Special Needs Families in the Military

Military Life

Military Life is a series of books for service members and their families who must deal with the significant yet often overlooked difficulties unique to life in the military. Each of the titles in the series is a comprehensive presentation of the problems that arise, solutions to these problems, and resources that are of much further help. The authors of these books—who are themselves military members and experienced writers—have personally faced these challenging situations, and understand the many complications that accompany them. This is the first stop for members of the military and their loved ones in search of information on navigating the complex world of military life.

1. *The Wounded Warrior Handbook: A Resource Guide for Returning Veterans* by Don Philpott and Janelle Hill (2008).
2. *The Military Marriage Manual: Tactics for Successful Relationships* by Janelle Hill, Cheryl Lawhorne, and Don Philpott (2010).
3. *Combat-Related Traumatic Brain Injury and PTSD: A Resource and Recovery Guide* by Cheryl Lawhorne and Don Philpott (2010).
4. *Special Needs Families in the Military: A Resource Guide* by Janelle Hill and Don Philpott (2010).

Special Needs Families in the Military

A Resource Guide

Janelle Hill and Don Philpott

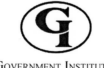

GOVERNMENT INSTITUTES
An imprint of

THE SCARECROW PRESS, INC.
Lanham • Toronto • Plymouth, UK
2010

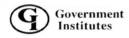
**Government
Institutes**

Published by Government Institutes
An imprint of The Scarecrow Press, Inc.
A wholly owned subsidiary of The Rowman & Littlefield Publishing Group, Inc.
4501 Forbes Boulevard, Suite 200, Lanham, Maryland 20706
http://www.govinstpress.com

Estover Road, Plymouth PL6 7PY, United Kingdom

British Library Cataloguing in Publication Information Available

Library of Congress Cataloging-in-Publication Data

Hill, Janelle.
  Special needs families in the military : a resource guide / Janelle Hill and Don Philpott.
     p. cm. -- (Military life)
  Includes index.
  ISBN 978-1-60590-715-4 (cloth : alk. paper) -- ISBN 978-1-60590-716-1 (electronic)
  1. Children of military personnel--Services for--United States--Handbooks, manuals,
etc. 2. Children with disabilities--Services for--United States--Handbooks, manuals, etc.
3. Families of military personnel--Services for--United States--Handbooks, manuals, etc.
I. Philpott, Don, 1946- II. Title.
  UB403.H55 2011
  355.1'2--dc22   2010034114

Contents

Foreword

The saying "It takes a village to raise a child" is especially true for families who have one or more children with special needs within the family. It takes an "army" of therapists, specialists, doctors, nurses, counselors, caregivers, educators, and other "helpers" to make a difference in the lives of these children.

From personal experience, the one light in my devastation over learning the vast injuries and damage done to my daughter, who was severely brain injured (hypoxic at birth with a failure to perform an emergency C-Section) and medically unstable due to prescribed pharmaceutical drug toxicity was a specialist in the Intensive Care Unit who told our family to "never bet against a child"; that their systems and brains have the greatest capacity to heal, and that love, stimulation, and appropriate care can make a tremendous difference. What I want to provide people as a result of our very painful and difficult journey is some insight into what persistence, determination, and resourcefulness can do in terms of making a vast difference in the quality of a child's enjoyment of life and ability to function at the highest possible levels of their individual capabilities.

This is not intended to be a guide for any specific special need, but an overall "compass" of sorts to help families familiarize themselves with their options. It is my greatest hope that some information within this guide can educate or inspire other families to leverage and maximize any and all resources available to provide the best possible opportunities to help children with special needs.

Note: While this book is primarily for families with children with special needs, reference is occasionally made to other family members who might also have special needs—returning wounded warriors, or spouses suffering from depression or addiction. However, this is not the focus of this book. Those who want to learn more about caring for wounded warriors should consult *The Wounded Warrior Handbook* (also by the authors of this book) which is dedicated to this subject. It is available at many libraries, and can be purchased at all leading bookstores.

Janelle Hill

Preface

This book was written to help all military families with special needs. Such families include those with children with physical or learning disabilities, a returning wounded warrior requiring long-term care, or an elderly relative who can no longer live independently. While the book focuses on families with special needs children, many of the benefits and services available to them are also available to adults with special needs.

The book begins with an overview chapter written for those parents who have just learned that their child has special needs. It focuses on the first steps that must be taken to get the help needed, and stresses that aid and support is always available so that one should never feel alone.

Subsequent chapters deal in more detail with matters such as health care, education, benefits, and so on. Throughout the book, we focus on how to act as your child's advocate, especially in matters of health care, treatment, and education. You have certain rights, certain services available to you, and certain avenues to appeal decisions that you think are unfair. All of this is explained in great detail.

Finally there is a comprehensive resource section that will enable you to get in touch with organizations and groups that can provide the support and resources you need.

ACKNOWLEDGMENTS

The authors would like to thank all the people who generously gave of their time to assist us with this endeavor. Much of the information that we have used comes from federal and military websites and is in the public domain. These include the Department of Defense, American Forces Press Service, U.S. Army Medical Department, Department of Veterans Affairs, Department of Health and Human Services, and websites of all branches of the U.S. military. We have tried to extract the essentials. Where more information might be useful we have provided websites and resources that can help you.

1

First Steps

With a population of 1.5 million active duty military members, each day around the globe, there are an estimated 540,000 active duty sponsors, each caring for a family member with special medical or educational needs. Most of those family members are children.

SPECIALIZED TRAINING OF MILITARY PARENTS

Specialized Training of Military Parents (STOMP) is the only National Parent Training and Information Center for military families providing support and advice to military parents without regard of the type of medical condition their child has.

STOMP (Specialized Training of Military Parents) is a federally funded Parent Training and Information (PTI) Center established to *assist military families who have children with special education or health needs.* STOMP began in 1985. A project of Washington PAVE (Partnerships for Action Voices for Empowerment), it is funded through a grant from the U.S. Department of Education. The staff of the STOMP Project are parents of children with disabilities who have experience in raising their children in military communities and traveling with their spouses to different locations.

STOMP serves families in four main ways:

1. By providing information, training, and workshops about laws, regulations, and resources for military families of children with disabilities
2. By connecting families to other families

3. By assisting parents and professionals in developing their own community parent-education/support group
4. By providing a voice to raise awareness of issues faced by military families of children with disabilities

For military families of children with disabilities, *STOMP is a one-stop shop for information and training regarding special education and other resources.* STOMP is a Project of Washington PAVE, a grassroots parent-directed organization. This combination brings together:

- Expert, comprehensive knowledge on disability/special education laws, rights, regulations, and responsibilities as they pertain to military families
- A wealth of personal experience and a network of personal contacts
- A parent-driven approach

Parents of children with special needs face many challenges:

- Feelings of isolation and anxiety
- Difficulty navigating disjointed services
- Severe financial worries
- Inadequate information
- Tremendous personal and marital stress
- Insurance bureaucracy
- Limited or no personal or private time
- Living in "survival mode"

These challenges are compounded when the family concerned is military. While all military families face certain challenges such as frequent Permanent Change of Station (PCS) moves or times when the military member is being placed in harm's way such as during wartime deployments, families with special needs family members face additional difficulties. For example:

- Continuity in provision of Individualized Education Program (IEP) services when moving from state to state or from state to DoDDS (Department of Defense Dependent Schools) overseas and DDESS (Domestic Dependent Elementary & Secondary Schools). In the United States, the Individuals with Disabilities Education Act (IDEA) requires public schools to develop an IEP for every student with a disability who is found to meet the federal and state requirements for special education. The IEP must be designed to provide the child with a Free Appropriate Public Education (FAPE). "IEP" refers both to the educational program to be provided to a child with a disability and to the written document that describes that educational program. At the end of twelfth grade, students with disabilities will receive an IEP diploma if they have successfully met the IEP goals. If they have met the requirements for the high school diploma, then the IEP diploma is not awarded.

- Availability of military member to be present to participate during IEP meetings/ medical treatments/procedures
- Finding specialists/physicians at a new duty station or location who will take TRICARE (military health entitlement program) and who are willing to accept new patients
- Re-establishing relationships with key medical and educational personnel in a new location
- Re-establishing eligibility for community resources to assist the special needs family member, as well as facing waiting lists for services needed
- Identifying within each state the array of services available and differences from state to state
- Differences in implementation of TRICARE services across the regions
- Lack of proximate family and community support due to geographical separations/time differences
- Additional financial burdens due to certain allotments and aspects of military pay calculations when considering eligibility (i.e., clothing allowance, separate rations, housing)
- Challenges with overseas assignments, i.e., denial of command sponsorship for family member with special needs (command sponsorship is necessary for eligibility for medical/educational systems), increasing family separations
- Difficulty implementing aspects of the Individuals with Disabilities Education Act (IDEA) because of host country agreements, i.e., transition services into vocational programming, community access, provision of related services
- Certain laws, regulations, and services that do not apply in overseas assignments, such as Section 504 of the Rehabilitation Act, the Department of Education regulations for the implementation of IDEA, and Medicaid
- Lack of local community support due to the self-containment/isolation/ military installations, and existing relationships between installation and local community

SPECIAL CARE ORGANIZATIONAL RECORD (SCOR)

The Department of Defense (DoD) has two very useful organizing tools for military families with special needs: the **Special Care Organizational Record (SCOR)** for Children with Special Health Care Needs and the SCOR for Adults with Special Health Care Needs. The SCORs are tools for caregivers, providing central repositories for recording and tracking information about their family member's ongoing support and health needs. Although the focus for each SCOR differs, they share the same fundamental goal of making it easier to organize, track, and update information for special needs family members.

The SCOR has multiple uses. It is designed as an organizing tool for families who have family members with special health-care needs. Use the SCOR to keep track of information about your family's health and care.

In caring for your family members with special health needs, you may receive information and paperwork from many sources. This organizational record helps you organize the most important information in a central place. The SCOR makes it easier for you to find and share key information with others who are part of your family's care team.

For example, families can use their SCOR to:

- track changes in medicines or treatments
- list telephone numbers for health-care providers and community organizations
- prepare for appointments
- file information about health history
- share information with primary care doctors, school nurses, daycare staff, and other caregivers
- review the checklist prior to making a PCS move

Each SCOR is tailored to the unique needs of a special needs family member. For example, the SCOR for Children includes sections for copies of a child's Individualized Family Service Plan or Individualized Education Program paperwork. The SCOR for Adults has sections for documenting daily routines, vacation preferences, employment and vocational experiences, and more. Each tool was vetted by the Exceptional Family Member Program managers, medical and education professionals, and the recognized disability expert, Dr. Ann Turnbull.

SCOR for Children with Special Health-Care Needs

Some helpful hints for using your child's SCOR:

- Keep the SCOR where it is easy to find. That way it will always be on hand when you need it.
- Be mindful that your SCOR contains very private information and that it should be kept in a safe place.
- Keep the SCOR as up-to-date as possible. Add new information to the SCOR whenever there is a change in a child's medical treatment.
- Keep the SCOR with you at appointments and hospital visits so that information you need will be close at hand.

How do you set up your child's SCOR? Follow these steps:

STEP 1: Gather information you already have.
Gather any health information that you already have about your child. This may include reports from recent doctor's visits, immunization records, a summary of a recent hospital stay, this year's school plan, test results, or informational pamphlets, etc. If you have a case manager with TRI-CARE, this individual may be able to help you gather that information.

STEP 2: Look through the pages of the SCOR.
Select the pages that you think will be most beneficial to you in tracking your child's health and care. Once you have determined what you need, print out those selected pages.

STEP 3: Decide what information is most important to keep in the SCOR.
What information do you find yourself looking for often? What information do your care providers need when caring for your child? Additional, less critical information can be stored in a file drawer or box where you can find it if needed.

STEP 4: Put the SCOR together.
Organize your SCOR in a way that makes the most sense to you and your child. Here are some supplies that may help you put it together:

- 3-ring binder or large accordion envelope to hold papers securely
- Tabbed dividers for creating separate sections
- Pocket dividers for storing reports
- Plastic pages for storing business cards and photographs

Things to remember about the SCOR:

- While the SCOR does contain a lot of your child's medical history/information, it is not intended to replace official medical records.
- It contains very private information (e.g., Social Security numbers, insurance information, medical history). It is imperative that you keep it in a safe place.

SCOR for Adults

The Special Care Organization Record (SCOR) for Adults is specifically designed as an organizing tool for families with an adult member with special health-care needs. This includes spouses and adult children with special health-care needs as well as any other adult dependent family member. The SCOR for Adults is intended to help track and organize information in one central location and to make it easier for someone to care for your family member when you are unable to do so. You can download your own copy from websites such as www.militaryonesource.com.

While the SCOR is organized in different sections, you are encouraged to reorganize it to accommodate your needs. Please note that while the SCOR for Adults is a tool kit to help you care for your family member, it is not legally binding in any way nor can it take the place of official medical records. It also contains very private information such as Social Security numbers, medical history/information, and insurance information. In order to ensure that you maintain your family's privacy, make sure to keep your SCOR in a safe place that is not easily accessible by those who should not have access to it.

How can the SCOR help you? While caring for your family member with special health needs, you receive information and paperwork that must be readily accessible. The SCOR will help you organize all of this information and make it easier for you to quickly find what you need. It will also make it easier for you to share key information with those who are part of your family member's care team.

Use the SCOR to:

- Track changes in your family member's medicines or treatments
- List telephone numbers for health-care providers and community organizations
- Prepare for appointments
- File information about your family member's health history
- Share new information with your family member's primary doctor and others providing care

Review the checklist prior to making a permanent change of station (PCS) move.

Some helpful hints for using your family member's SCOR:

- Keep the SCOR where it is easy to find. That way it will always be on hand when you need it.
- Be mindful that your SCOR contains very private information and that it should be kept in a safe place.
- Keep the SCOR as up-to-date as possible. Add new information to the SCOR whenever there is a change in your family member's treatment.
- Keep the SCOR with you at appointments and hospital visits so that information you need will be close at hand.

How do you set up your family member's SCOR? Follow these steps:

STEP 1: Gather information you already have.
Gather any health information that you already have about your family member. This may include reports from recent doctor's visits, immunization records, a summary of a recent hospital stay, test results, or informational pamphlets, etc.

STEP 2: Look through the pages of the SCOR.
Select the pages that you think will be most beneficial to you in tracking your family member's health and care. Once you have determined what you need, print out those selected pages.

STEP 3: Decide which information is most important to keep in the SCOR.
What information do you find yourself looking for often? What information do your care providers need when caring for your family member? Additional, less critical information can be stored in a file drawer or box where you can find it if needed.

STEP 4: Put the SCOR together.
Organize your SCOR in a way that makes the most sense to you and your family member. Here are some supplies that may help you put it together:

- 3-ring binder or large accordion envelope to hold papers securely
- Tabbed dividers for creating separate sections
- Pocket dividers for storing reports
- Plastic pages for storing business cards and photographs

Things to remember about the SCOR:

- While the SCOR does contain a lot of your family member's medical history/information, it is not intended to replace official medical records.
- It is not legally binding in any way. The SCOR provides a place to start thinking about who would take care of your family member if you were no longer able to do so. However, you would still need to go through the proper legal protocol to make these decisions legally binding.
- It contains very private information (e.g., Social Security numbers, insurance information, medical history). It is imperative that you keep it in a safe place.

CHILD DEVELOPMENT SYSTEM

Frequent family separations and the requirement to move, on average every 3 years, place military families in situations not often experienced in the civilian world. For military families, finding affordable, high quality child care is paramount, if they are to be ready to perform the mission and their jobs. It is also important to military personnel that child care services be consistent and uniform at installations throughout the military.

Both the Army and Marine Corps have implemented a process to determine and review the best placement and support for children with special needs in the child care setting.

Army Special Needs Accommodation Process (SNAP)

In the Army, the Special Needs Accommodation Process (SNAP) is carried out by a subcommittee of the installation Exceptional Family Member Program (EFMP) committee. The core team membership consists of the installation EFMP manager, Children and Youth Services (CYS) coordinator, Army public health nurse and parents, augmented, as appropriate, with CYS program staff, CYS school liaison officer, school personnel, staff judge advocate representative, family advocacy program manager, and other medical personnel.

The installation EFMP manager assumes or designates a chairperson of the team. The team will:

1. Explore child care installation and youth supervision options for children/youth that have a medical diagnosis that reflects life-threatening conditions, functional limitations, or behavioral/psychological conditions.

2. Determine child care and youth supervision placement considering feasibility of program accommodations and availability of services to support child/youth needs.
3. Recommend placement setting that accommodates to the extent possible the child's or youth's individual needs.
4. Develop and implement DA Form 7625-3 (SNAP Team Care Plan).
5. Conduct annual periodic review of the child/youth individual SNAP Care Plan and/or, as requested, by CYS.
6. Establish an installation SNAP Review Team consisting of garrison commander or designee, staff judge advocate, installation EFMP manager, and CYS coordinator. The Review Team will be available, on request, to ensure that a SNAP Team has explored all options for reasonable accommodation.

Marine Corps Special Needs Evaluation Review Team (SNERT)

In the Marine Corps, the SNERT is a team of qualified personnel whose goal is to make an assessment of the accommodations necessary for a special needs child to participate in Marine Corps Children, Youth, and Teen Programs (CYTP) and determine the most appropriate placement for the child.

Installation SNERT teams report to the installation commander and shall include, but not be limited to the following members:

• CYTP Administrator
• EFMP Coordinator
• Medical personnel
• Parent(s) of child
• Child or youth, when appropriate
• Other applicable CYTP or community agency personnel

Additional information about the Marine Corps SNERT can be found in Marine Corps Order P1710.30E, "Marine Corps Children, Youth and Teen Programs," 24 June 2004.

TRANSITIONING / MOVING

Moving is an integral part of life as a military family. There are belongings to pack, a move to plan, expenses to be tracked, and a new home to find. When a family has a child with special needs, these experiences are even more complicated and emotion-filled.

Resources

As part of the military community, there is a lot of help available, such as financial help for the move and, if desired, a sponsor waiting to help at the new duty station. It will benefit the entire family to take advantage of these resources.

The Exceptional Family Member Program

It is mandatory in the military that a dependent with special needs, whether a spouse or child, be enrolled in the Exceptional Family Member Program (EFMP). To enroll in EFMP, contact the Family Support Center at the nearest military installation. This will ensure that your child's medical and educational needs will be considered as a duty station is selected. Service members will be assigned to an area where their EFM's educational and medical needs can be met, provided there is a valid personnel requirement for the service member's grade and specialty.

Service members have the option of accepting assignments where services for EFMs do not exist. Choosing this option usually means that the service member must live apart from the family so that the EFM can continue to have his or her needs met. Contact the EFMP office at the new duty station to let them know that you are coming and what your family's needs might be. If respite care or specialized daycare is needed, the EFMP coordinator can help suggest available resources.

Family Support Centers

Once you know you are moving, contact the nearest Family Support Center and ask to speak with a relocation specialist. The Relocation Assistance Program offers a wealth of information for the relocating service members and their families. Be sure to discuss your moving allowances and understand how they are computed. This is also a good place to look for resources to help meet the needs of an exceptional child. The Family Support Center can also connect you to the Exceptional Family Member Programs and to available respite care programs. To find a family center near you go to www.militaryinstallations.dod.mil.

Plan My Move

PlanMyMove (planmymove.mhf.dod.mil) is a comprehensive moving tool that lets you create customized moving tools such as calendars, to do lists, and arrival checklists, all intended to help you get organized and to make your next move as smooth as possible. It includes tools for military families with special needs.

Schools

Ask your child's current teacher to write a letter introducing your child to the new teacher. An overview of what the teacher sees as strengths and weaknesses, as well as a description of what works well with your child will help the new teacher. Contact the new state's Parent Training and Information Center (www.taalliance.org) for information on schools in the new area.

Medical Concerns

Before moving, check to see what medical care is available at the new duty station. The Provider Directory on the TRICARE website (www.tricare.mil) can help locate specialty services. Phone numbers are listed so that providers can be contacted in advance to be sure that they are still network providers and are currently accepting new patients.

If a child has special physical needs, take extra care to ensure that the child's records are kept safe. Before moving, make copies of the child's important documents and leave copies of papers with grandparents or close friends if possible. Consider checking out the medical record from the existing duty station and delivering it personally to the new duty station. If this is not allowed, request a full copy of any and all medical records prior to the transfer in the event the record becomes lost or incomplete in transit.

Tell the Kids

For some families, the news that the family is moving is best presented at a family meeting. If you think the reaction is likely to be positive, this is probably a good idea. If, however, you think your kids are going to be upset, it may be a good idea to tell them one on one before the family meets to discuss this. This will allow time to react to each child individually, and may avoid a scene where one upset child sets the tone and then negatively influences the other children.

> Before telling the kids about the move, arm yourself with some of the positive aspects of your new home: Is it closer to friends or family? Are there beaches? Is it near an amusement park?
>
> If your kids are old enough, show them your new home on a map and begin the discussion of your journey to your new home.
>
> Should your child have a special interest, find out if there is a museum on the way to your new home that your child would not be able to experience otherwise.

Decide the best way to present the move and give thought to how you will handle various emotional responses.

Discuss ways your children can keep in touch with friends, or have a visit planned before you move away so the good-bye won't be so final.

Be positive. If you are upbeat about your move, your kids will be reassured that all will be well.

If your child has concerns, or is grieving for his or her old home already, it is very important that you show your child that you understand this sorrow, and that it is natural and normal. You might share some of your own sorrow coupled with some aspect of the new home that you are looking forward to.

Remind your child that the present home was once new, and yet they made friends. This will happen again.

A calendar or timeline with pictures of things that will be happening leading up to, during, and after the move may help calm the fears of younger or special needs children who rely on daily reminders to help them prepare for what each day will bring.

Have a family meeting to discuss the children's feelings, whether they are excited, angry, or worried. Reassure your children that all these feelings are normal.

Find time in normal rituals of meal preparation or bedtime to have one-on-one conversations with your children, so they can share their thoughts and feelings about the move.

Plan a farewell party. Take lots of photos and collect addresses, e-mail addresses, and phone numbers.

If your child is old enough, provide a scrapbook for the child to assemble.

Since many families now have Internet service on computers and phones, consider setting up a Google Gmail Video Chat, Apple iChat, or a similar web chat service so that friends and family can "visit" online. Using social networking applications such as Facebook or MySpace can also help connect loved ones and friends over long distances and help children remain connected, which is especially important during transitions and changes to routines.

Moving away from the familiar and into the unknown can be scary. Give your children opportunities to express their feelings. Happy and excited feelings are much easier to accept and deal with, but negative feelings, like sorrow or anger are just as valid. If your children feel that only happy thoughts should be expressed, the negative emotions will just go underground and may well surface as negative behaviors. This does not mean your child is entitled to set a negative tone for the whole family or that poor behavior is acceptable, but honest talk may diffuse some of the difficulty.

Packing

Before the movers arrive, set aside the following items in a room with a big sign on the door asking movers to stay out, or, to not pack:

> Important documents such as school records, dental records, any medical records, birth certificates, insurance policies, copies of PCS orders, and a copy of the household inventory form.
> Medicine and medical equipment that will travel with you.
> Comfort needs, like a pillow, favorite stuffed toys, or some favorite music or DVDs.
> Valuables such as jewelry, hard drives, laptops, and related personal items that will travel with you.

Also consider packing and labeling a few "first night" boxes. These boxes would contain sheets, plastic cups, plates and eating utensils, toilet paper, additional medical supplies or equipment, towels, extra toiletries, and other items that will help you settle in while the new residence is being unpacked and established. For young children, adding some special surprises like little books, toys, or games for first night unpacking can help as a needed distraction.

Overseas Suitability Screening

Before being stationed overseas or to a remote assignment, all families of service members are screened for overseas suitability. The screening is mandatory and used to determine if the member or family member(s) have any special needs that may require special medical or educational attention. The presence of a special need does not mean a family is ineligible to travel overseas; however, it does mean extra care may be necessary to be sure the family is living in an area that is suitable to all family members.

Traveling with Kids

Whether traveling by plane, train, or automobile, traveling with children takes some planning. The following tips will help make the trip go smoothly:

- Be sure to inform the Traffic Management Office (TMO) a child has special needs.

- Be proactive in contacting the airlines or other services to assure there are arrangements for wheelchair or other equipment storage, and to find out the locations of accessible bathrooms. If a wheelchair is needed at the gate, make the calls yourself to be sure this happens and double check at check-in to be sure the airline is fully prepared to support these needs.
- Keep security items within reach.
- Have healthy snacks at hand.
- Bring plastic bags for trash.
- Bring books, cards, and games to help pass the time. A few new items may hold a child's attention longer than an old favorite.
- A child might enjoy being in charge of his/her own travel bag; however, regulate how much is put into this bag so that it doesn't get too heavy!
- Bring an inexpensive umbrella stroller; these can be especially helpful in airports and train stations.
- Tape emergency contact information in children's clothing or have them wear a medical alert bracelet.
- Take a portable DVD player if possible, along with the child's favorite DVDs as well as comforting music for bedtime.
- Keep hand wipes ready for frequent hand cleaning after stops and before eating.

Air Travel

The Air Carrier Access Act prohibits airlines from prohibiting passengers on the basis of disability and actually requires U.S. air carriers to accommodate the needs of passengers with disabilities. For more information contact www.disabilityinfo.gov.

Keep the following things in mind as you prepare for the trip:

- Contact the airline 48 hours in advance of the flight if special services are needed, such as a respirator hook-up or transportation of an electric wheelchair.
- Ask if the bathrooms are accessible flying on an older or small aircraft.
- Remember that assistive devices do not count toward the limit on the number of pieces of carry-on luggage. Wheelchairs (including collapsible battery-powered wheelchairs) and other assistive devices have priority for in-cabin storage space (including in closets), as long as you take advantage of preboarding.
- Ask your physician about the safety of flying if a family member suffers from seizures. Get the physician's recommendation in writing and carry it with you as part of your family's medical records.

- Consider bringing a stroller to gate check, as there can be a lot of ground to cover between gates.
- Use a backpack instead of a diaper bag, as it will leave your hands free to hold on to kids.
- Bring snacks for the kids, as few self-respecting toddlers will eat airplane food, and on many flights only a small bag of pretzels is offered anyway.
- Decide if boarding early would be the best choice for your family. Air-conditioning is generally not turned on until just before take-off, so a squirmy child would have to remain still longer than necessary in an overheated plane. Some families tag team, with one parent boarding early with the bags and the other parent boarding later with the kids.
- Be sure the car seat you have is compatible with airline seats. Check the airline's website for car seat information.
- If you are traveling with a service animal, notify the airline in advance so arrangements can be made to seat you and the animal accordingly.
- Ensure that you have appropriate identification and boarding passes within easy reach for security.
- Ensure that any medicines that may qualify as liquids, aerosols, or gels are properly labeled as prescription or required medicines in order to pass through security.
- If hygiene items are required, pack 2–3 times the needed amount for carry-on, in order to accommodate additional airline delays that may be unexpected. The same goes for special foods or medications, in the event of an airline delay or cancellation that can cause up to an overnight delay.
- Sometimes the military will pay for first-class accommodations in the event that transporting an EFM requires the extra space, leg room, or ability to fully recline. If your doctor justifies it in writing, there is a process to get special approval for financial coverage of that requirement.

Traveling by Train

If you are traveling by train, Amtrak will assist those with wheelchairs in the case of high or low platforms or bi-level trains. Your child may remain in the wheelchair en route or the chair may be stowed. Should your child require oxygen, you must make reservations in advance and give notice of your need to bring oxygen on board at least 12 hours before you board. Please call 1-800-USA-RAIL (1-800-872-7245) for more information about bringing oxygen on an Amtrak train, as well as station accessibility.

Train travel means that more interaction with children is possible than in a car, especially if there is only one driver. Be sure to bring activities your child enjoys, such as favorite stories, card games, and healthy snacks. Many Amtrak trains now offer wireless Internet connectivity and electrical outlets at the seats so that DVD players, laptops, and phones can charge while traveling. Check to find out if your particular train service offers these features. Amtrak does sell a limited selection of meals, snacks, and beverages on their services; it is recommended that you check ahead of time to be sure that what they make available on the service meets any dietary restrictions of the EFM. If not, plan ahead to bring your own food. Also, trains can be delayed on the tracks just as easily as at time of arrival or departure. Sometimes trains can be delayed en route significantly. It doesn't hurt to pack some extra toilet paper, hygiene items, hand sanitizer, snacks, and items to pass more time than you may think you'll spend, just in case.

Traveling by Car

Traveling by car affords a family greater flexibility than by plane or train. You can stop and explore or stretch your legs when you would like to. To make the most of the journey, plan a route with places of interest to stop along the way. Provide children with a map with the route to the new home clearly marked, and stops along the way marked as well. Car games will help pass the time. Download a map of the United States (www.eduplace.com) and have the children color in a state each time they spot a license plate from that state. Have a scavenger hunt with each family member trying to spot items on a list.

In some cases, EFMs must travel by car for periodic stops, or to have a route that covers proximity to medical facilities en route. Other times, a single parent cannot drive long distance and travel with an EFM because the EFM may require monitoring and a medical attendant may be unable to travel with the adult. Many times driving is a full-time requirement, and the EFM's medical needs cannot be simultaneously attended to, or the drive depletes the energy of the adult, and the adult is ultimately too tired to also provide EFM care. Talk to the EFM's doctor and the command about this situation because in certain cases, the military will pay (or reimburse) to transport the automobile to the new duty station and provide alternate transportation to ensure the EFM's care remains the priority and that the care requirements and safety requirements are accommodated. This type of situation is evaluated on a case-by-case basis, though there are precedents already established for reasonable accommodations.

Temporary Lodging

For information about temporary lodging, go to www.military.com and click on "Travel" and then "Military Lodging Options." Make reservations as far in advance as possible. Mention your family's EFMP status, as some bases have special accommodations. Be sure to ask if they have wheelchair accessible rooms or rooms with TTY for the deaf or hearing impaired if necessary. Many **Morale, Welfare, and Recreation (MWR)** facilities also have special rooms for providing lodging with families traveling with service animals.

MORALE, WELFARE, AND RECREATION (MWR)

MWR in history started on the battlefields of World War I, where behind the lines, Salvation Army sisters and Red Cross volunteers ministered to the needs of soldiers as the forerunners of today's morale, welfare, and recreation specialists. After the war was over, funding stopped, and morale programs were mothballed. It wasn't until July 1940 that the Morale Division—later named Special Services—was established within the Adjutant General's Office.

Between 1946 and 1955, the core recreation programs were established and staffed by a combination of active duty military and civilians. Until the mid-1980s, active duty enlisted personnel held military occupational specialties in Special Services and were assigned at every level of command. As those occupational specialties were discontinued, civilians continued to operate MWR programs with military oversight. Special Services underwent much reorganization and had many names before coming to its present configuration as MWR.

Some families find the time in transit, while waiting for belongings to catch up with them, to be a bit of a break from the usual household responsibilities. When there is only a suitcase of clothes, the amount of work necessary to keep up the family is diminished. Take this time to find fun in the new area. Help kids to enjoy themselves and get a positive feel for their new home.

Housing

Should your family live on base or off? Five percent of on-base housing has the advantage of being wheelchair accessible, a feature that can be hard to find off base. Life on base has the added advantage of other military families close by. Becoming part of a supportive community may be easier on base than it is off, where neighbors may not understand or be interested in the military lifestyle. A big factor in this decision is the wait for housing, which varies from base to base. Some services offer priority housing to eligible families with EFMs. If there are special housing requirements or accommodations necessary for an EFM, such as installing pocket doors or railings, the base housing office can work with the EFM's medical documentation and physicians to provide certain modifications where they are deemed medically necessary. This is evaluated on a case-by-case basis.

Schools

An important factor in your decision about housing is schools. Investigate both on-base, if available, and off-base schools. Contact these schools well in advance of the move to begin the discussion of how your child's unique needs will be met. Meet with administrators of both systems to share your child's Individualized Education Plan (IEP), and see what is available in each system. Your child's IEP should be honored until a new IEP is written, but available services may vary, as might the individual school's approach to special education. Even on a base with a DoD school, the child might be transferred off-base if it is determined that the civilian school is better suited to the child's needs. This is more likely if the child has severe or profound challenges. Schools, both on-base and off-base, develop reputations in the existing military special-needs community. Sometimes contacting a local educational advocate's office is a good idea because advocacy groups are often hired to participate in support of negotiating IEPs for families. The **Marine Corps Special Needs Evaluation Review Team (SNERT)** and Military One Source can help you locate advocacy groups in your area. WrightsLaw (www.wrightslaw.com) is also a good source for referrals and connectivity in new communities. Those groups will know which schools have a reputation for providing a quality, free, and appropriate education versus those that tend to be less enlightened about the implementation of the Individuals with Disabilities Education Act (IDEA). Some schools and/ or their districts use legal due process to "slow roll" military families out of their district in an attempt to save money and conserve resources, which is not in the child's best interests. Advocates will know which schools or districts have a reputation for this and can prevent placement in undesirable or less-appropriate programs. Schools use a rating system to determine levels of disabilities of children and part of that rating system involves a mathematical calculation of additional funds a district may provide to a school to implement services for that child. It is important to know what your child's rights and entitlements are, as well as have a connection to someone who understands how those calculations work, in order to know how to negotiate for services for your child. For instance, your child may be eligible for curbside pickup at a residence or care facility and may require an air-conditioned bus if sensitive to heat sickness or seizures. Your child may need vision therapy, physical therapy, or occupational therapy as deemed educationally appropriate for acquiring a relevant or particular set of skills. Perhaps a Least Restrictive Environment (LRE) needs to be discussed and selected. Perhaps specific, measurable, qualitative, and quantitative goals need to be established in order to determine progress during the increments of the school year, with regard to academic, behavioral, and similar categories of instruction. Perhaps your child needs an individual aide, or may need to share access to an aide. Perhaps your child would significantly regress if not continued in a similar services–program during the summer break that other children take. Special needs are individualized and therefore so are IEPs. So it is incredibly important for parents to be informed, educated, and prepared to advocate for their children, because the school's first priority is to their budget, not to your child, and therefore the best interests of the child must be represented by the parent and often an informed companion advocate. Advocates for hire can be very expensive, but many work with community agencies and grant programs to offset their costs, and others are experienced parents who volunteer to participate and assist.

Child Care

For working parents, finding high-quality care is a high priority. As a military parent of a special needs child, finding child care that can accommodate shift work, extended hours, and weekend duty and can meet the unique needs of a child can be challenging.

Look for child care that is inclusive. Inclusive child care allows children to learn together in an educational atmosphere that supports and nurtures the individual strengths of each child, and each child participates in the daily routines and activities of the class regardless of cognitive or physical impairments. Every child deserves the opportunity to interact with other people regardless of his or her ability level.

Most military installations have special resource teams to help parents of special needs kids find appropriate child care. These teams may comprise child care specialists, an EFMP advocate, a public health nurse, and the parents. The purpose of this team is to explore child care and youth activities for children with certain special needs who are involved in installation child care or youth programs. The team will identify the care options available to best meet the child's needs as well as consider any increased technical support, special services, or staffing that may be necessary to care for the child appropriately.

For more information about child care, check with the installation's Resource and Referral Office. A resource specialist can guide you through the registration process, accreditation and fees, and the exploration of both on- and off-base options to choose the best care for your child. Installations have different names for the office that manages the child care programs, so if the name of the office is unknown, the best place to start is at the home installation's Child Development Center (CDC): ask which office provides local child care resource and referral services. Telephone numbers of all CDCs and school-age programs can be found at www.militaryhomefront.dod.mil/efm.

It is possible for a base child development center to inform you that they cannot provide care for your EFM under certain circumstances. In this case, the EFM Coordinator and the command should continue to work with the family in order to identify in-home or related appropriate care. It is important that when selecting a duty station, that this issue be explored ahead of time because it can happen that a base can accommodate the EFM but not the child care center, and ultimately the military parent has a conundrum because care is not guaranteed. Try to work preventatively to ensure this does not happen.

Questions to Ask about Child Care

What are the priorities for placement on the list at this installation?

I have more than one child. What is your policy on placing siblings?

What process do you use for keeping my data up-to-date?

Will you get in touch with me, or will I be responsible for periodically updating you?

What is the range of time that I might have to wait for a space to open up in my child's age group?

My child is an EFM and I am on deployment status with a pending departure date, does this impact priority placement for my child?

I will need child care during the interim. Will you help me find it?

What is your child/provider ratio?

Will the center adapt the physical environment to meet my child's needs with the goal of increasing his or her participation?

Will the providers adapt materials and curriculum to promote independence and capitalize on my child's favorite activities?

Do the providers have experience working with adaptive devices?

What types of training have the providers had?

How will the center implement and monitor my child's IFSP or IEP?

Will the center allow me to work with the care providers to show proper positioning, use of equipment, medication administration, etc?

Will therapists have a quiet area to work with my child?

How will the center facilitate diapering? (Sometimes centers will not have changing tables or rooms for 3- and 4-year-olds, let alone much older children requiring support with Activities of Daily Living [ADLs].)

Do you have staff members who know American Sign Language (ASL) or have experience working with augmentative communication devices?

What are your emergency medical procedures? How close are they to a medical facility? Do you have a nurse on staff?

Does the center have a discipline policy? (Ask for a copy.)

Does the center have a method for filing complaints? Whom would I speak with?

Do you provide Emergency Respite Care?

Do you have someone on staff qualified to administer prescription medications? What are your policies on providing emergency medication, such as for onset of seizures or allergic reactions?

Is this a peanut- or other nut–free facility?

If food or beverage is provided to the EFM during the day by the facility, with whom can we review all ingredient labels to ensure our EFM is not accidentally exposed to a dangerous ingredient?

Moving In

Move-in day is exciting. The new house starts to feel like home, and everyone is relieved to have familiar objects back. Give thought to creating moving-day traditions. They can be as simple as having Chinese take-out the first night in a new home, or eating the first meal on boxes, even though the table is back. Because of the excitement, pay special attention to children who may wander or find danger in unfamiliar surroundings. If respite care is needed, contact the family support center ahead of time to prepare to have help well in advance.

Safety in a New Home

Look over a new home with an eye for hazards such as busy roads or creeks nearby. Hold a family meeting to discuss these hazards with children and establish firm boundaries defining where they are allowed to go. In some cases, base housing or certain apartments and condominium associations can post signs for hearing- or vision-impaired family members to help neighbors and travelers realize extra precautions must be taken in the area, such as for a "deaf child at play."

If a child is likely to run away from the house, talk to the neighbors, local police, the local fire department, and/or the Military Police (MPs) about this. Provide them with a current photo and a description of the child. Explain how the child is different and might react if confronted. Be sure to include all contact information on the sheet and give copies to the MPs or local police. Remember to update the photo and contact information as necessary. List any medications and/or diagnoses that can impact first responders' approaches and knowledge of volatile situations. You may want to make several copies of this to have on hand in case of emergency and to take with you when you travel.

If you are concerned that despite much vigilance a child may leave the house unobserved, consider installing extra locks, barriers, or an alarm system. Ask your physician for a letter explaining the medical necessity for these modifications and bring it along with a request to the base housing office or landlord to ask permission to install extra locks.

Talk to neighbors about concerns for your child. Give them your phone number and ask them to call if they spot your child moving away from the house alone. If a child is deaf or blind, contact the base or local authorities and ask for a sign alerting drivers to the presence of a deaf or blind child.

If oxygen tanks are in the home, the local fire department needs to know about them. Also, if a child is likely to hide in the case of an emergency, tell the fire department. A copy of the child's ID page that was made for the police would be appropriate for the fire department as well.

If a child is not verbal, consider keeping identification and contact information on the child, perhaps on a bracelet or sewn into clothes.

It is recommended that signs for pets, service animals, and identifying disabilities be posted by the front door or in a visible window to alert first responders in an emergency.

SPOUSE EMPLOYMENT

Frequent relocation, extended deployments, and other unique aspects of the military lifestyle can create significant career and employment challenges for military spouses. Having a special needs child brings even further challenge. You may desire employment due to financial necessity or to fulfill personal goals. Fortunately, there are resources available to assist you.

Military Spouse Career Center

To enhance employment and career opportunities for military spouses, the Department of Defense partnered with Monster.com to develop the Military Spouse Career Center. This virtual resource found at www.military. com/spouse can provide assistance to you regardless of your location. The center was created to provide career-networking services, employment services, and information to military spouses. The center provides information on spouse-friendly employers, education and scholarships, licensing and certification, job search skills, and much more. The center enables employers to post jobs for military spouses at no cost. Additionally, military spouses can create and post resumes and explore thousands of job openings around the world.

MilitaryHOMEFRONT (www.militaryhomefront.dod.mil) also has information on spouse employment in the "Troops and Family" section.

Installation Support

Many installations have a family support center that offers professional family member employment readiness training and support services. Installation-based employment assistance programs provide job search training and assistance and serve as a source of information for local job fairs and job search databases. Training and other support services for spouses may include the following:

- Resume writing
- Skills assessment
- Career interests assessment
- Access to computers and the Internet
- Individual counseling and career planning
- Job search skills
- Information about local job listings
- Career seminars
- Support and encouragement

DEPLOYMENT

Waiting for a loved one to deploy is hard on children as well as spouses. Children may not understand why a parent must leave and may fear the parent is leaving forever. Because children are not very good at expressing their worries verbally, they tend to express them behaviorally. Be sure your children have many chances to express how they are feeling. The following ideas may help your family prepare for and get through a period of separation due to deployment:

Use your own words to help children find theirs. For example, "I don't want Daddy to leave, and waiting for him to leave makes me feel sort of sad and worried. Do you ever feel that way?"

Explain that although many things will be different, many things will be the same.

If the child plays imaginary games with dolls or animals, try to introduce the idea of one member of the doll family leaving. Let the other dolls say how they feel about this.

Use a map or a globe to show where the child's parent will be.

Use a calendar to show children when the deployment will take place, as they may not understand how long three weeks is. Some families cross a day off the calendar, others count with buttons or M&Ms from a jar.

Be sure that the departing parent has time with each child before deploying. Hug often. Take photos of each child with the departing parent. Sometimes a parent will go to "Build A Bear" and get a recording of their voice installed in the paw, so the child can squeeze it and hear a short, loving message from the parent. Others video-record stories, loving messages, and songs for their children to hear while they are away. Photos can also be placed on everything from mugs, to t-shirts, blankets, and pillowcases, which can help children have something to enjoy and share as a keepsake during the absence.

The departing parent might schedule a trip to the child's school to meet with the teacher. The point of this trip is to be sure the teacher knows about the change in the family dynamics. Let the child show you around his or her school world and perhaps hear you tell the teacher how proud you are of him or her. You will be able to ask better questions about your child's day if you are familiar with his or her school. Many schools can Skype, i-Chat, or otherwise virtually assist the deployed parent to participate in IEP meetings and school communications; often many are willing to do so if asked with time to pre-plan.

Have a family meeting about ways to keep in touch during the deployment. Letters, pictures, tapes, and movies are all good ways to stay connected. Communications and "care packages" should also come from the child to the parent, so they remain engaged and involved, if possible.

Remember to occasionally send children their own letters. Children enjoy few things more than receiving their own mail! A letter to the family pet will also bring a smile to a child's face.

Find the best way for the child to mark the end of the deployment. This may be making Xs on the calendar or ripping links off a paper chain.

Remember that just because a child doesn't express his or her feelings, it doesn't mean they are not troubled. If a child is acting out, it may be the result of unexpressed emotions. Help the child name these feelings.

It is fine and even healthy for children to see you have sad feelings too, but if you are really about to fall apart, try to do this away from your kids. Strong emotions in a parent can be scary to a child.

Remind children that they are still safe and that a deployed parent is still a member of the family.

Do not minimize the child's grief. To a child it may feel like a parent is lost forever. Grief without understanding is difficult to work through.

Children may often punish the parent there for the disappearance of the parent who is not there; and often the deployed parent is not aware of major behavioral changes that occur after their departure. Parents must be prepared for the potential of "acting-out" behavior because of anger, frustration, sadness, and confusion.

Help Is Available

If you or your children are having a particularly difficult time adjusting to the deployment, counseling is readily available through several sources. Call the family service center or contact www.militaryonesource.com. Through TRICARE you are entitled to eight sessions of counseling without a referral from your Primary Care Manager. If more is needed, an authorization can be obtained. Another source of support may be a chaplain. It is important to ask if the chaplain is licensed for marriage or family therapy. The parent at home has a heavy load to carry. As a parent of a disabled child, things can be difficult enough when both parents are available, but now it may seem overwhelming. Taking care of yourself has never been more important. Do not hesitate to contact your EFMP coordinator to ask for respite care. The entire family will benefit if the parent at home has the chance to recharge his or her batteries.

Coming Home

When the deployed parent returns, children may feel worried and stressed, as well as happy and excited. Depending on the child's developmental level, he or she may feel uncomfortable around the returning parent, almost as if they were strangers. For some children, even good change is unsettling. Remind your returning spouse of this and help him or her understand that the child's behavior is a reaction to change, and not a rejection of the returning parent. Returning parents must also understand that routines are important and they have not been part of the routine for some time. Transition and adjustment to the returning parent can be stressful and cause the child (and the spouse) anxiety. Returning parents are certainly excited to come home to their families, but should be careful to integrate back into the home environment safely and with appropriate readjustment for all family members. Returning parent: your spouse has been "running the show" without you for some time, and they've probably figured out what works. Respect it and respect them. Offer help and ask your spouse how he or she feels it is best to reintegrate and participate.

Make sure children have time to let their excitement out with the returned parent before having quiet time with your spouse. However, once the excitement has subsided, do schedule time to reconnect. Maintaining a strong marriage is one of the best things parents can do for their children. Returning parent: your spouse may have been "single parenting" an EFM, multiple EFMs, or an EFM plus other children. As much as your return requires adjustment on everyone's part, the spouse that has been "single parenting" for an extended period is going to need a break just as badly as you need a break from that deployment or departure. It is important to make sure both parents get down time for an extended period of time upon someone's return, as much as possible. This "down time" may be as simple as time for an uninterrupted hot bath, or uninterrupted sleep, or time to go to the gym. Make sure both parents get this uninterrupted time for each individual's mental, physical, emotional, and spiritual health.

DISASTER PREPAREDNESS

Families with special needs must be prepared for evacuation or other emergencies. Careful preparation will reduce stress and hardship. Remember that more time may be needed to evacuate.

You may want to include the following when packing for an evacuation:

- 30 days' supply of medication and prescriptions
- Copies of all prescriptions
- Important documents (medical records, insurance papers, birth certificates, and veterinary documents such as for service animals)
- Enough diapers and clothing for 7 days
- Bed rail
- Special eating utensils
- Special food or groceries, which disappear quickly when the supply chain to a region is disrupted

- Entertainment for children (e.g., games, cards, books)
- Comfort items such as blankets or toys
- Battery-operated flashlight and radio, with extra batteries
- A current photo and physical, behavioral, and medical description of your child including a list of necessary medication
- Contact information for your child's physician
- Water
- Hand sanitizer and hygiene items
- Cash and credit cards with no balance on them for emergencies
- Any supplies for an assistive animal, such as a crate, food, water, bowls, litter, medicines, and jackets, leashes, or harnesses
- A back-up hard drive with PDFs of records, photos, and important information
- The location, contact information, directions, and any other information related to shelters that are set up for disabilities (You can pre-register with the county to identify your EFM's special needs so that they are prioritized and documented as needing evacuation in an emergency.)
- A way to charge your phone from your car or a spare battery if electricity is not readily available
- A map and two detailed sets of directions for two alternate ways to evacuate an area, with some information about where the family can go
- If there is a "hurricane" season or a time when evacuation may be anticipated, be sure the automobile has adequate fuel and service, and that some supplies are pre-organized for rapid departure.
- Prepare a list of e-mail addresses or phone numbers to store so that in the event of an emergency, you can contact others and they can reach you.

Service Animals

Federal law allows service animals into emergency shelters. In your packet of important papers be sure to include the animals' rabies tag and license. The license must not be expired. Service animals may need to be registered with your county of residence and may also need to be registered with the base. Remember that in a disaster, the service animal may become confused or distressed and may need more attention than usual. Handlers of service animals must be wary of working animals experiencing distress because even well-trained animals have survival instincts and can experience fear and react in extreme situations. Many people do not understand they are supposed to act indifferently toward working animals and may attempt to approach, pet, or play with working animals. It is important that handlers of working animals communicate and advocate not just for the EFM, but for the animal's rights, welfare, and safety also. In many states the minimum penalty for interference with a working animal of a disabled person is a misdemeanor charge. Know your state laws and have a printout of your state's statute (often conveniently kept in the crate or in a zippered pouch of a working jacket) so that you and your animal's rights are protected.

Service animals must have the appropriate records to document their training and certification as a working or service animal at all times. If emergency medical care is required for a service animal, given proof that the animal is a working animal, many veterinarians deeply discount the cost of their services because the animal dedicates its life to service of an individual in need. If the animal is a working animal that wears a jacket or has a collar, including contact information on the handler and the EFM can help first responders identify and reconnect a service animal and a family that are accidentally separated in an unforeseen event. Microchipping is also recommended for this purpose.

Power Loss

In times of disaster, extended power outages may last for weeks. If you live in military housing and require electricity for vital medical equipment, contact the EFMP coordinator or housing manager. If generators are not available, contact the Primary Care Manager to discuss whether your child should be moved to a hospital or other facility where power is available. Vital medical equipment may range from monitors to respiratory support equipment. For even short power outages due to a storm, ensure that you have adequate power back-ups so that basic care can continue under any circumstances.

Transition to Adulthood

Between the ages of 14 and 16, a child's IEP will begin to address the transition process to adulthood. During transition planning, students and their families find out about community agencies and programs that provide services to persons with disabilities after high school. Some of these adult services include job training and placement, assistance in getting housing, and programs on health care and independent living. These transition services should start no later than the first IEP to be in effect when the child turns 16, and should be updated annually thereafter. Also, no later than 1 year before reaching the age of majority under state law, a child must be informed of his or her rights under IDEA, if any, that will transfer to him or her upon reaching the age of majority. Remember to include an older child in the IEP process.

In some cases, programs may start earlier with counseling to help an EFM transition to puberty and set expectations for physical changes as well as developmental changes that precede adulthood.

Parents should investigate eligibility for Social Security, disability, and related services that a child may be ineligible for until they reach 18 years of age.

Independent Living

As a parent, you began teaching self-help skills very early in your child's life. Self-advocacy skills are also important. Whenever possible, let the child speak for himself or herself. This might be encouraging a child to order his or her own food in a restaurant or to explain to a new teacher his or her need to tape record lessons.

The time to begin thinking about assisted living facilities is when a child is young, as the waiting lists can be years long. Contact the state you will retire to and inquire about what services are available.

One of the most important adult services, vocational rehabilitation, is available in most states. Vocational rehabilitation services include planning, assistance, support, and training that help a person get ready for and find a job. Contact the state's Parent Training Center, www.taalliance.org, and ask about programs that help with transition.

It important to remember that unlike special education services, vocational rehabilitation services are not automatically available to a person with disabilities. A person must meet certain qualifications, and some agencies also charge fees for their services. Because there is no central system of adult services as there is for special education, it may be necessary to deal with an assortment of adult services and government programs.

If you as a military member or spouse are retiring or aging during this time when your child must be prepared for assistive or independent living, you may want to consult with an attorney who specializes in Special Needs Trusts, and consider establishing a special needs trust rather than a will, which may provide funds or resources for the EFM during your lifespan and thereafter, while avoiding probate laws at the time of death of the parent. This type of preparation can ensure that transitions to adulthood and provisions for ongoing care during adulthood for an EFM are well planned and well executed.

CARING FOR YOUR ADULT CHILD

Parents of healthy children can usually plan on their children living independently and becoming financially independent. However, if your child has a lifelong disability you will need to plan not only for childhood care, but adult life as well, even if only to help with "executive functions" like paying bills or making certain decisions. Will the child be able to make decisions about health care or finances? For an adult child to qualify to receive Supplemental Security Income or Medicaid, he or she cannot have more than $2,000 in assets. So how can you ensure a child's well-being and financial security?

Supplemental Security Income (SSI) and Medicaid

The Supplemental Security Income program provides a minimum monthly cash payment for categorically aged, blind, and disabled individuals. Eligibility is based on the limitation of assets and should not be confused with other Social Security benefits. Medicaid is frequently tied to SSI approval and a program to pay for health care for certain low-income or disabled individuals or families. Medicaid does not pay money to you; instead, it sends payments directly to health-care providers. Depending on the state's rules, it may be necessary to pay a small part of the cost (co-payment) for some medical services. Many states have special Medicaid programs for people with disabilities, and not all are income based.

The Special Needs Trust

Special Needs Trusts are discretionary trusts created for people with disabilities to supplement, but not replace, public benefits. This type of trust will allow a disabled individual to continue to receive SSI, Medicaid, Section 8 housing, and other public programs while benefiting from trust fund money. The money from this trust can be used to purchase special wheelchairs, handicapped accessible vans, as well as to pay for vacations, a personal attendant, or recreational and cultural experiences. SSI is designed to pay for food, clothing, and shelter. Medicaid will pay for medical bills. The trust fund can be used for all other needs that are identified in the trust document. Contact a lawyer who has experience with Special Needs Trusts. Don't hesitate to act because of concerns about paying for the service. Make some calls and explain your situation. Many lawyers will consider reducing their fees or allowing payment on a monthly basis for their services. If you think you do not have the assets needed to fill a trust, remember that life insurance is an asset, as is a home if you own it. Trusts can hold property and other assets, not just cash. Compared with wills, which can be contested, trusts are a valuable way to avoid probate, significant cost, and time lapse. There are different kinds of special needs trusts, such as for personal assets or for litigation proceeds.

A Special Needs Trust, sometimes called a Supplemental Needs Trust, is a specialized legal document designed to benefit an individual who has a disability. There are three main types of special needs trusts: the first-party trust, the third-party trust, and the pooled trust. All three name the person with special needs as the beneficiary. A "first-party" special needs trust holds assets that belong to the person with special needs, such as an inheritance or an accident settlement. A "third-party" special needs trust holds funds belonging to other people who want to help the person with special needs. A "pooled" trust holds funds from many different beneficiaries with special needs.

Another trust is a D4A Trust, which gets its name from Federal Law, Section 136p(d) (4) (A). The trust is established for the lifetime benefit of an individual under age 65 who is either blind or disabled as defined by the Social Security laws, and requires that at the beneficiary's death, the state will be repaid for all Medicaid the beneficiary received during his or her lifetime. The trust may only be established by parents, grandparents, courts, or guardians, not by the disabled individual directly. The "D4C" pooled trust is similar, but may be established directly by the individual. The D4C pooled trust account may pay any remaining funds to the nonprofit organization that holds the trust, rather than (or as well as) to the state, but no funds may pass to other beneficiaries.

Letter of Intent

This letter provides parents with an opportunity to speak to whoever will be caring for and making decisions for their child after they have died. This may be the person who is the trustee for the Special Needs Trust. You may want to write out your child's story in the letter, including medical history and educational background. Describe the child's favorite activities, foods, and people. Include places he or she has gone, and places he or she would like to visit. This tool will help whoever is taking care of your child to better know you and your child. It will provide information to help them understand your wishes and expectations as they make decisions about your child's future.

Guardianship and Declaration of Incapacitation

Usually, when a child turns 18, it is assumed that he or she is capable of making decisions about health, finances, and the future. Once your child turns 18, you will no longer be able to talk to your child's physician about his or her health. You will have no control over financial decisions or contracts your child might sign. If you are concerned that a child will not be capable of making these decisions responsibly, consider asking the courts for guardianship.

Guardianship is a court-approved relationship between a legal guardian and a person with a disability. The court defines the degree of legal authority that a guardian will have to act on behalf of the disabled person. Detailed documentation from a physician will be needed to show that your child is not mentally capable of becoming independent. Be aware that if you move to another state, it may be necessary to apply for guardianship in the new state.

ID Cards for Adult Children

Unmarried children of military sponsors who are age 21 and over, severely disabled, and are disabled due to a condition that existed prior to the child's 21st birthday are entitled to TRICARE benefits. These adult children are eligible to retain their military ID cards as well. In the Navy and the Marine Corps, this program is called The Incapacitated Dependents Program; in the Army the program is called Incapacitated Children Over 21.

Army families can call:
317-510-2774/2775
Navy families can call:
910-874-3360
USMC families can call:
703-784-9529/30
If you are retired or a former spouse, call 1-800-336-4649
Air Force families can call:
210-565-2089

HOSPICE CARE

Hospice care is available for terminally ill patients and their families when the patient has been given a terminal, life-limiting prognosis. The goal of Hospice care is to provide dignity and comfort to the dying. Eighty percent of hospice care occurs in homes or nursing homes, and TRICARE will cover most of the costs.

If you live on base and your child is in hospice care, arrange a meeting with the Military Police, your chaplain, and your EFMP coordinator. This will help ensure all parties understand your wishes for your child. This is very important, as without this meeting, well-meaning but misguided Military

Police or emergency response personnel may insist on trying to resuscitate your child against your wishes.

Checklist for Your Special Needs Child

- ☐ Passports, visas (be sure to write down the numbers and keep them in a safe place)
- ☐ Wills
- ☐ Copy of medical records
- ☐ Individualized Family Service Plan (IFSP)
- ☐ Individualized Education Program (IEP)
- ☐ Individual Habilitation Plan (IHP)
- ☐ Dental records
- ☐ Service members' Group Life Insurance (SGLI) Election Form
- ☐ Social Security cards (be sure to write down the numbers and keep them in a safe place)
- ☐ Copy of Family Care Plan
- ☐ Copy of EFMP enrollment paperwork
- ☐ Child Care Plan
- ☐ Registration for child/daycare
- ☐ List of important numbers
- ☐ Insurance policies pertinent to your child (auto, home, life)
- ☐ Inventory of household goods and stored property pertinent to your child
- ☐ Service animal records
- ☐ Birth certificates
- ☐ Adoption papers
- ☐ Death certificates
- ☐ Divorce papers as they pertain to your child (custody agreement)
- ☐ Shot records
- ☐ Contracts and loans
- ☐ Citizenship/naturalization documentation
- ☐ Auto club membership cards/information
- ☐ I.D. cards
- ☐ Warranties for equipment
- ☐ Federal and state income tax records
- ☐ Copies (several) of TDY and PCS orders
- ☐ Diplomas/transcripts
- ☐ Power of attorney
- ☐ Special needs trust of a member whose parent is deploying in wartime

The following should be completed prior to deployment:

- ☐ Update Emergency Data Card in Military Personnel Record and get copies
- ☐ Establish/arrange joint checking/savings account (write down all account numbers and keep them in a safe place)
- ☐ Identify available emergency services
- ☐ Ensure parent/care provider knows how to make contact in case of emergency
- ☐ Renew Armed Forces I.D. Cards
- ☐ Review information related to Red Cross/Service Relief Societies
- ☐ Identify and resolve problems with cars, household, and appliances
- ☐ Share information related to Military Family Support programs
- ☐ Identify Medical Facilities, TRICARE, and CHAMPOS
- ☐ Establish family budget and resolve any family business issues
- ☐ Make copies of orders (at least 10 copies of PCS orders)
- ☐ Complete a security check on the house

It is recommended that both parents sign and obtain a passport for the child before the parent deploys, because an individual parent cannot obtain one without the other's signature. They may also both need to be present in order to obtain an ID card for the child with the local DMW because a single parent may not be able to obtain the card if their spouse is deployed.

EXCEPTIONAL FAMILY MEMBER PROGRAM (EFMP)

More than 100,000 military families have members with special needs. These include spouses, children, or dependent parents who require special medical or educational services. These family members have a diagnosed physical, intellectual, or emotional condition.

The Military Services use the term "Exceptional Family Member Program (EFMP)" to refer to a program with two different functions: a personnel function and a family support function.

The EFMP personnel function:

- Is a mandatory program for all active duty service members.
- Is standard across all Services.
- Identifies family members with special medical and/or educational needs,
- Documents the services they require, and
- Considers those needs during the personnel assignment process (especially when approving family members for accompanied travel to overseas locations).

- Involves the personnel and medical commands and the Department of Defense educational system overseas.

The EFMP family support function:

- Is not mandatory. DoD policy on family centers allows, but does not require, the Military Services to offer family support services to exceptional family members within the Military Services' family support systems.
- Differs from Service to Service.

The Exceptional Family Member Program (EFMP) serves these families in several ways (see table 1.1).

The Army and the Marine Corps staff their family centers with individuals whose responsibility is to provide support to families with exceptional family members. They are called the EFMP Managers (Army) or EFMP Coordinators (Marine Corps).

In the Navy, the EFMP staff who support the personnel function may also provide family support services, but the Navy does not staff their family centers with EFMP Coordinators.

Table 1.1

Service	Support Service	Provider
Army	Family Support	Installation EFMP Manager Location: Army Community Service (ACS)
Army	Personnel Function	Special Needs Advisor Location: Medical Treatment Facility
Marine Corps	Family Support Personnel Function	EFM Coordinator Location: Marine Corps Community Services (MCCS)
Navy	Family Support	Information and Referral Specialist Liaison to the EFMP Fleet and Family Support (FFS)
Navy	Personnel Function Family Support (limited)	EFM Coordinator Location: Medical Treatment Facility
Air Force	Family Support	Airman and Family Readiness Center (A&FRC), formerly the Family Support Center. Please visit the Airman and Family Readiness Flight website for more information.
Air Force	Personnel Function	Exceptional Family Member Program (EFMP) Reassignment and Humanitarian Reassignments. Please visit the Air Force Crossroads website for more information.

Air Force Exceptional Family Member Program (EFMP)

The Air Force's Exceptional Family Member Program (EFMP) is designed to provide support to military family members with special needs. EFMP Services includes a variety of personnel, medical, and family support functions. The Exceptional Family Member Program—Family Support (EFMP-FS) is the community support function provided by the Airman and Family Readiness Centers (A&FRCs) that includes, but is not limited to, on- and off-base information and referral, parent training, support groups, relocation assistance, financial management, and school information.

Enrollment Categories

Category I: Needs do not generally limit assignments. Enrollment for monitoring purposes for medical or educational needs.

Category II: Limited overseas/remote continental United States (CONUS) assignments. Care is usually available at most locations, except for some isolated CONUS/overseas areas. If orders are for overseas duty, the family must successfully complete overseas screening.

Category III: No overseas assignments. The medical or educational condition precludes assignment to overseas locations based on nonavailability of medical and/or educational services at most overseas locations.

Category IV: This medical or educational condition requires assignment to billets near major medical treatment facilities within the continental United States only.

Category V: This category includes a provision for homesteading in an area where the service member can fulfill both sea and shore duty requirements, typically in the geographic areas of Norfolk, Jacksonville, San Diego, Bremerton, and Washington, D.C. Eligible families are those having an EFM with multiple/severe disabilities or medical problems, or highly complex educational requirements.

Category VI: (Temporary category) The medical or educational condition requires a stable environment for six months to a year due to ongoing treatment of diagnostic assessments. Must be updated in 1 year to receive permanent category or to be disenrolled.

Air Force Special Needs Identification and Assignment Coordination (SNIAC)

The Special Needs Identification Assignment Coordination process (SNIAC) provides medical information management support for EFMP enrollment functions, and coordinates relocations for families who have medical or educational needs. Both EFMP-FS and SNIAC work together with EFMP-

Assignments at the Air Force Personnel Center (AFPC) to provide comprehensive and coordinated medical, education, and community support; assignment coordination; as well as housing accommodation to families enrolled in the EFMP program.

The SNIAC process identifies eligible U.S. Air Force families with special medical and/or education requirements and helps those families obtain required services. This SNIAC process ensures those families have access to necessary services upon reassignment, whether CONUS or OCONUS.

The SNIAC process identifies sponsors whose family members have special needs for reassignment purposes. The SNIAC process assists the Military Personnel Flight (MPF) in updating the Assignment Limitation Code Q that is assigned to the sponsor for the purpose of ensuring availability of medical and/or educational services upon PCS. Therefore, SNIAC enrollment is mandatory for active duty sponsors whose family members meet enrollment criteria established by DoD and U.S. Air Force policy. The SNIAC helps families connect with medical and educational programs with the goals of increasing family self-sufficiency and improving family self-advocacy skills

The Air Force Special Needs Coordinator (SNC) and Family Member Relocation Clearance Coordinator (FMRCC) are typically located in the Life Skills Support Center and/or Family Advocacy office at the Medical Treatment Facility (MTF).

The SNIAC process is not a standard family support center program within the Air Force. To locate SNIAC personnel and receive more information please visit the Air Force Special Needs website. **Please note**: At this time, this information requires a Common Access Card (CAC) PKI certification for access.

Army Exceptional Family Member Program

The Army Exceptional Family Member Program (EFMP) is a mandatory enrollment program implemented through AR 608-75. EFMP, working in conjunction with other military and civilian agencies, provides a comprehensive, coordinated, multi-agency approach for medical, educational, and community support; housing; and personnel services to families with special needs. The Army EFMP includes both personnel and family support functions.

Personnel Function

Enrollment allows assignment managers at Army personnel agencies to consider the documented medical and special education needs of EFMs in the assignment process. When possible, Soldiers are assigned to an area where their

EFMs medical and special education needs can be met. This will depend on a valid personnel requirement for the Soldier's grade, specialty, and eligibility for the tour. All Soldiers are still eligible for worldwide assignment.

Enrollment in the EFMP is mandatory for Active Army Soldiers, U.S. Army Reserve (USAR) Soldiers in the USAR-Active Guard Reserve (AGR) program, and other USAR Soldiers on active duty exceeding 30 days, and Army National Guard (AGR) personnel serving under authority of title 10, USC.

Soldiers are responsible for keeping their EFMP enrollment current as an exceptional family member's condition changes or at least every three years, whichever comes first.

Family members must be screened and enrolled, if eligible, when the Soldier is on assignment instructions to an area outside the continental United States for which command sponsorship/family member travel is authorized and the Soldier elects to serve the accompanied tour. This screening consists of a review of medical records for all family members and developmental screening for all children 6 years and younger.

Enrollment in the EFMP does not adversely affect selection for promotion, schools, or assignment. Information concerning enrollment in the EFMP or any of the data used in the program is not made available to selection boards.

Soldiers who are members of the Army Married Couples Program must both enroll in the EFMP when they have a family member that qualifies.

Enrollment Criteria

Criteria for enrollment are contained in AR 608-75, Appendix B.

Identification Process

Early identification: Early identification aids Army personnel agencies in considering the special medical and/or educational needs of the family member early in the process of identifying a future assignment. Early identification aids the Soldier and family members in avoiding late and costly approval of overseas accompanied travel. Early identification can be achieved:

- During routine medical care by the health-care provider at the military treatment facility
- During completion of in-processing and out-processing query sheets by the soldier
- By self-identification by the Soldier or family member

Overseas screening: All Soldiers with assignment instructions for outside the continental United States who elect to serve the accompanied tour must have family members medically and educationally screened and, if required, enrolled in the EFMP. This process should be completed within 30 days of receipt of assignment instructions. Identification during overseas screening can result in a delay of approval for the family member travel if the family member has a special medical or educational need and has not been enrolled in the EFMP previously.

When are family members screened? Family members are screened when the Soldier is on assignment instructions to an area outside the continental United States for which command sponsorship/family member travel is authorized and the Soldier elects to serve the accompanied tour.

The steps in the process are:

- Soldier is placed on assignment outside the continental United States.
- Military Personnel Division personnel service battalion verifies family members' eligibility for accompanied tour.
- Soldier receives authenticated DA Form 5888 (Family Member Deployment Screening Sheet) for screening and DA Form 4787-R (Reassignment Processing) for reassignment processing.
- Military treatment facility screens family members for medical and/or educational needs.
- The Soldier/spouse completes DA Form 7246 (EFMP Screening Questionnaire) and signs and authenticates DA Form 5888.
- *If no medical or developmental problems are identified* in the screening process, block 9a is checked to indicate that EFMP enrollment is not warranted. NO FURTHER EFMP ACTION.
- *If a family member requires further evaluation,* DD Form 2792 (Exceptional Family Member Program Medical Summary) and/or DD Form 2792-1 (Exceptional Family Member Special Education/Early Intervention Summary) are completed.
- *If enrollment is warranted,* the forms are forwarded to the appropriate regional medical command for coding.
- The regional medical commands enroll eligible Active Army Soldiers into the program. The Army Reserve Personnel Command and the Army National Guard enroll eligible Reserve and Guard personnel. The date that DD Form 2792 and/or DD Form 2792-1 is sent for coding is entered into block 9b of DA Form 5888.
- Military Personnel Division/personnel service battalion coordinates with the gaining command to determine if services are available.

- Military medical makes recommendations on locations where medical services are available.
- DoD Dependents Schools identifies pinpoint locations where educational needs can be met (if applicable).
- Housing office indicates availability of housing.
- When services are not available at the location to which the soldier has been assigned, Army personnel agencies consider alternative assignment locations based on existing assignment priorities or, upon approval of the appropriate authority, send the Soldier on an unaccompanied tour.

   o Deletion from assignment instructions is not granted solely because of a Soldier's enrollment in the EFMP. The EFMP is designed to be an assignment consideration, if Soldier is enrolled, and not an assignment limitation. Soldiers could be reassigned to an "all others tour" to meet Army requirements.
   o Deferment for Soldiers with family members enrolled in the EFMP is granted when family travel decisions from the gaining command are not finalized.

EFMP Personnel Points of Contact

Special Needs Advisors are the points of contact for initiating enrollment in the EFMP. The Special Needs Advisors are located at military treatment facilities.

Family Support Function

AR 608-75 requires installation of Exceptional Family Member Program managers. These individuals are located in Army Community Service (ACS) centers.
   The installation EFMP managers:

- Advises the installation commander and supported troop commanders of EFMP issues that affect their Soldiers.
- Serves as chair of the installation EFMP committee and, at a minimum, conducts meetings quarterly. If the committee is not in existence, submits appropriate documents to the installation commander to establish such a committee. The committee may be a subcommittee of the Human Resource Council.

   o Provides comprehensive minutes to the installation commander for approval and furnishes a copy to the military treatment facility commander.

o Maintains approved minutes on file under file number 608-75a and destroys minutes when no longer needed for current operations.

o Includes, at a minimum, representatives from Army Community Service, military treatment facility, Military Personnel Division/ personnel service battalion, civilian personnel advisory center, directorate of public works, staff judge advocate, child and youth services, community recreation, public affairs office, and schools. One or more representatives who are exceptional family members or parents of an exceptional family member are invited to participate when appropriate.

• Establishes a special needs resource team as a subcommittee of the installation EFMP committee and serves as a member of the special needs resource team, and assumes or designates a chairperson of the team. The special needs resource team:

o Explores child care and youth activities options for children with special needs in installation child and youth programs.

o Determines child, youth, and family care options for care and activities considering feasibility of program accommodation and availability of technical support.

o Recommends placement that accommodates, to the extent possible, the child's or youth's individual needs and parent mission requirements and preference for care/activity setting.

o Performs secondary functions of technical support and the need for increased staff/provider support.

o Makes referral to special education/services, and conducts periodic placement review of children enrolled in installation child and youth programs.

o Members, in addition to the installation EFMP manager, include the community health nurse, child and youth services coordinator, other program managers who work in the care/activity setting in which placement is being considered, and parents of the child. The team can be augmented by the child's primary medical care provider, psychologist, assigned social worker, therapists, or early intervention program personnel as appropriate. Other health care professionals may provide consultation.

• Coordinates care for the child/youth, as part of the individualized family service plan or the individualized educational program, with the special needs resource team.

• Participates in in-service and ongoing professional training.

- Submits annual EFMP budget request to the ACS director.
- Develops an installation EFMP standing operating procedure.
- Tracks installation EFMP participants using documents provided by military treatment facility EFMP staff, Military Personnel Division/personnel service battalion, and other authoritative sources.
- Updates the EFMP section of the DA Form 3063 (Army Community Service Management Report).
- Assesses relocating soldier's EFM housing and community support needs (for example, Army Community Service, child and youth services, and community recreation) prior to departure. Shares required service information with the gaining installation EFMP manager (continental United States) or MACOM EFMP manager (outside the continental United States), who notifies the affected installation agencies prior to EFM's arrival.
- Assists families in developing solutions to individual and community EFM issues and problems (for example, inaccessible facilities and programs) and informs and advises the installation commander of EFM needs.

USMC Exceptional Family Member Program

The Exceptional Family Member Program (EFMP) is a mandatory enrollment program mandated by Marine Corps Order P1754.4A, Exceptional Family Member Program for all active duty personnel. The program provides assistance to service personnel with family member(s) who have special needs before, during, and after relocation due to Permanent Change of Station (PCS) orders.

In the Marine Corps, the EFMP has two functions:

Personnel Function (Assignment Coordination): To identify, enroll, and coordinate with personnel on accompanied travel for family members who have exceptional needs. The primary goal is to ensure the special needs of the Exceptional Family Member (EFM) can be met at a new assignment location. EFMP enrollment information enables Marine Corps Occupational Field Monitors to proactively consider a family member's special needs requirements during the assignment process and to pinpoint the assignment to a location with appropriate resources that address the special needs. Successful implementation requires up-to-date enrollment information and extensive coordination among the personnel, medical, and educational communities.

Family Support: To coordinate the EFMP at the installation level—assist families and the command with issues related to the exceptional family member.

Personnel Function

Policy. The EFMP provides for assignment of Marines with family members who have special needs to locations where those needs can be met. Operational requirements of the Marine Corps and requirements for career development and experience are considered in making assignments. Final responsibility lies with the sending Commanding Officer and Navy Medical officials to ensure each Marine is accurately screened prior to assignment and qualified for reassignment. The following policies apply:

1. ACCOMPANIED ASSIGNMENTS—OVERSEAS. These will not be affected if the required medical services are available at the overseas location. It is imperative that the EFM's needs be formally re-evaluated if the sponsor considers extending his/her overseas assignment or if he/she is being considered for reassignment to another overseas location. Overseas screening is the same for all families anticipating accompanied orders overseas.
2. ASSIGNMENTS—UNITED STATES. Permanent Change of Station (PCS) assignments within the continental United States, Alaska, and Hawaii will be approved if the exceptional needs of the family member can be met in the proposed assignment area or the appropriate director, CMC (Manpower Management Division), or CMC (Reserve Affairs) determines that the needs of the Marine Corps take precedence.
3. The EFMP has no impact on the deployment responsibilities of the sponsor. Overseas unaccompanied, unit deployments, and standard deployments must be carried out without interruption. When the family's needs conflict with such assignments, the assignment will be affected under the provisions of a humanitarian transfer.
4. Marines having EFMs will not normally be assigned to accompanied tours in geographic areas where another military department is responsible for providing medical and medically related services. When necessary, appropriate coordination will be conducted by CMC (MHF) with the department to verify the availability of the required service.
5. The sponsor will always have the option of accepting assignments where medical services needed by the EFM do not exist, while the EFM is supported in another location.
6. Enrollment shall not adversely affect advancement, career potential, or eligibility for special programs and assignments.

Eligibility criteria. An exceptional family member is defined as an authorized family member (spouse, child, stepchild, adopted child, foster child, or a dependent parent) residing with the sponsor who may require special medical or educational services based on a diagnosed physical, intellectual, or emotional handicap such as asthma, cerebral palsy, mental retardation, dyslexia, attention deficit disorder (ADD), attention deficit disorder/hyperactivity (ADHD), autism, oppositional defiant disorder, or depression. Disabilities may range from mild to severe.

Enrollment process.

- Ensure your family member is enrolled in DEERS.
- Contact your EFMP Coordinator at Marine Corps Community Services, who will assist you in obtaining medical and educational evaluations, and provide the necessary forms for you, your medical provider, and, if necessary, your child's school official to complete.
- Return the completed forms to the EFMP Coordinator, who will forward them to the appropriate Central Screening Committee and to Headquarters Marine Corps for processing and category assignment.
- The U.S. Navy Central Screening Committees (health-care providers) evaluate EFMP enrollment packages and assign a category to each exceptional family member based on the individual's needs and reflecting limitations to an assignment. The categories are:

  o Category I—EFM's needs generally do not limit assignment.
  o Category II—EFM requires pinpoint assignment overseas and within CONUS.
  o Category III—EFM can have no overseas assignments.
  o Category IV—EFM requires location in major medical areas in CONUS.

- DD Form 2792, Exceptional Family Member Medical Summary and DD Form 2792-1, Exceptional Family Member Special Education/Early Intervention Summary are used by all of the Military Services in the enrollment process.

EFMP Coordinators located at Marine Corp Community Service centers assist families in both enrolling in the EFMP and assist families in navigating the system. In the enrollment process, the EFMP Coordinators:

- Initiate enrollment for EFMP referrals.
- Assist sponsors in obtaining medical and educational evaluations.
- Forward completed EFMP enrollment forms to the appropriate screening committee.

- Maintain copies of enrollments and care management notes in files until EFMP families PCS to a new duty station.
- Ensure confidentiality and security of EFMP case files.
- Educate local commands and communities of EFMP issues.
- Notify local unit commanders of enrollment and category of sponsors in that unit.
- Advise sponsor when a family care plan should be developed.
- Maintain a central registry of EFMs.
- Generate a quarterly installation roster.

In addition the EFMP Coordinator will assist you with locating and identifying:

- Local support groups
- Points of contact for:

  o State and National Parent Training Centers
  o Protection and Advocacy groups
  o TRICARE Region and local TRICARE Service Center
  o Local school district special education offices, to include the Department of Defense schools
  o Local recreation for special needs children and adults
  o Special programs, services, and adaptations that are unique to the local installation and surrounding community

Family Support Function

The necessity of frequent moves can make it difficult for exceptional families. It takes time to get the correct services in place for the family member with disabilities, and with each move, families must begin again. The EFMP Coordinators located at Marine Corp Community Service centers assist families in navigating the system. In this capacity, the EFMP Coordinators serve as advocates for local EFMP activities and issues and as a link between exceptional families.

EFMP Coordinators provide families with information about:

- Local support groups.
- Points of contact for:

  o State and National Parent Training Centers
  o Protection and Advocacy groups
  o TRICARE Region and local TRICAREService Center

- o Local school district special education offices, to include the Department of Defense schools
- o Local recreation information for special needs children and adults
- o Information about any special programs, services, and adaptations that are unique to the local installation and surrounding community

Points of Contact

Marine Corps Headquarters (Personal and Family Readiness Division). EFMP manager is responsible for:

- Managing EFMP applications and screening committee eligibility notifications.
- Notifying sponsors of enrollment by letter.
- Ensuring regional and installation EFMP Coordinators are notified of enrollment and category of sponsor.
- Interfacing with Commandant of the Marine Corps (CMC) (Manpower Management) and CMC (Reserve Affairs) to pass enrollment information.
- Coordinating and submitting EFMP resource requirements through budget channels.
- Sponsoring training workshops, publishing regulatory guidance, and providing consulting services to EFMP Coordinators regarding program policies and procedures.

Exceptional Family Member Program Manager
Personal & Family Readiness Division (MR)
Headquarters, U.S. Marine Corps
Quantico, VA 22134-5103
Commercial: 703-784-9654
Toll Free: 1-866-464-6110
EFMP Coordinators

- Located in Marine Corps Community Service centers
- Assist families in enrolling in the EFMP
- Provide support services
- Manage the installation EFMP for the Commander

Regulations

EFMP guidance is contained in:

- SECNAV Instruction 1754.5B, 14 December 2005, Exceptional Family Member Program
- BUMEDINST 1300.2A, 23 June 2006, Suitability Screening, Medical Assignment Screening, and Exceptional Family Member Program (EFMP) Identification and Enrollment
- MCO P1754.4A, 10 April 1997, Exceptional Family Member Program

Navy Exceptional Family Member Program

The Navy's Exceptional Family Member Program (EFMP) is designed to assist Sailors by addressing the special needs of their exceptional family members (EFM) during the assignment process. Special needs include any special medical, dental, mental health, developmental, or educational requirement, wheelchair accessibility, adaptive equipment, or assistive technology devices and services.

In the Navy EFM program, the primary function is the personnel function. The Navy EFMP Coordinators are located at the medical treatment facility, not at the Fleet and Family Support Centers (all Fleet and Family Support Centers have an EFMP liaison). The Navy EFMP Coordinators serve both personnel and family support functions, but with an emphasis on the personnel function.

Personnel Function

The goal of the EFMP is to ensure the special needs of the EFM can be met at a new assignment location. EFMP enrollment information enables Navy detailers to proactively consider a family member's special need requirements during the assignment process and to pinpoint the assignment to a location with appropriate resources that address the special needs. Successful implementation requires up-to-date enrollment information and extensive coordination among the personnel, medical, and educational communities.

EFMP enrollment is mandatory and required immediately upon identification of a special need. DD Form 2792, Exceptional Family Member Medical and Educational Summary and DD Form 2792-1, Exceptional Family Member Special Education/Early Intervention Summary are used for enrollment. DoD civilian employees and their family members do not enroll in the EFMP.

Command points of contact and Navy medical treatment facility (MTF) EFMP coordinators can assist service and family members with the enrollment process.

Sailors may be reluctant to enroll because of misconceptions that EFMP enrollment may limit assignments and career advancement, or preclude family members from accompanying sponsors on overseas tours. These negative perceptions are not supported by fact. Sailors enrolled in the EFMP have always received equal consideration for accompanied assignments and for promotions.

Eligibility criteria.   Special needs include any special medical, dental, mental health, developmental or educational requirement, wheelchair accessibility, adaptive equipment, or assistive technology devices and services.

Enrollment process.   Special needs are:

- Identified during routine health care (Medical Treatment Facility or TRI-CARE Health Provider)
- Self-identified (service or family member)
- Identified during Suitability Screening by the Suitability Screening Co-ordinator

Next Steps

Refer the service and family member to the Medical Treatment Facility EFMP Coordinator who assists with completing DD Form 2792-1, Exceptional Family Member Special Education/Early Intervention Summary, DD Form 2792, Exceptional Family Member Medical and Educational Summary, and required addenda as follows:

1. The MTF EFMP Coordinator forwards the completed enrollment form to the appropriate regional Central Screening Committee (CSC). CSCs are located at Naval Medical Center Portsmouth, San Diego, and U.S. Naval Hospital, Yokosuka, Japan.
2. The CSC reviews the enrollment form, recommends a category code, and forwards the form to the Navy EFMP Manager (PERS-45) in Millington, Tennessee, or to HQ USMC EFMP in Quantico, Virginia.

There are six Navy EFMP enrollment categories:

- Category I—for monitoring purposes only
- Category II—pinpoint to specific geographic locations
- Category III—no overseas assignments
- Category IV—major medical areas in CONUS
- Category V—homesteading
- Category VI—temporary enrollment—update required in 6–12 months

3. PERS-45 confirms the category code and enters the enrollment data into an EFMP data base.

Navy detailers use the EFMP enrollment data to pinpoint assignments to locations with appropriate resources that can address the special needs.

NOTE: If you are going to have receipt of orders in the next nine months, begin to update now to avoid unnecessary delays.

EFMP Coordinators, located at Navy medical treatment facilities:

- Provide necessary EFM forms DD 2792.
- Assist staff and sponsors in the application process.
- Forward completed EFMP enrollment forms to the appropriate screening committee.
- Maintain copies of EFM enrollment files and ensure confidentiality and security of EFM case files.
- Forward applications to Navy EFM Central Screening Committee.
- Maintain liaison with other MTF EFMP Coordinators and overseas screening offices.
- Coordinate with Fleet and Family Support Centers to provide EFMP training, as necessary, to all area commands.
- If serving at an overseas MTF, provide liaison with the DoD schools and the other Military Services having responsibility for medically related services to ensure required services are available.
- Develop and maintain an EFMP central database that reflect the local area EFMs
- Interact with the Health Benefits Advisor and the TRICARE Area Case Manager to coordinate required medically related services.
- Maintain working liaison with the Navy Personnel EFMP Manager to identify emergency enrollments.

Family Support Function

The Navy EFMP Coordinators are located at the medical treatment facilities. Their role in the family support function is to refer enrollees to the Fleet and Family Support Center EFMP Liaison for community assistance.

Points of Contact for the EFMP

Headquarters/personnel. Navy Personnel Command (NAVPERSCOM) in Millington, Tennessee, is the proponent for EFMP. Contact information for the EFMP Operations is (901) 874-4390; DSN 882-4390 or via E-mail. Contact information for the EFMP Policy (N135) is (901) 874-6670; DSN 882-6670 or via E-mail.

NAVPERSCOM is responsible for:

- Prescribing EFMP enrollment and disenrollment procedures.
- Coordinating detailing procedures including those for severely disabled EFMs.
- Prescribing procedures for expeditious screening and forwarding of EFM forms from the sponsor or MTF via the Central Screening Committee to the EFMP Manager.
- Establishing and maintaining a database of enrolled service members with EFM.
- Establishing and maintaining a current EFM resource database that includes medical, educational, and support agencies, facilities, and services in key fleet concentration areas.
- Developing and periodically conducting training and information campaigns.
- Providing relocation assistance.

Headquarters/Edical. Bureau of Medicine and Surgery (BUMED) in Washington, D.C., also has EFMP responsibilities. BUMED contact information is (202) 762-3451; DSN 762-3451 or E-mail.

BUMED and Navy MTFs are responsible for:

- Developing policy for health-care providers and patient administrators to identify and enroll eligible family members in the EFMP.
- Maintaining Central Screening Committees comprised of health-care providers who review completed EFMP applications and recommend disposition to NAVPERSCOM.
- Identifying an EFMP coordinator at each Navy MTF who will assist staff and service members with the application process and provide necessary enrollment forms.
- Providing training, as necessary, to all area commands on the EFMP.
- At an overseas MTF, coordinating early intervention, special education, and medically related services with the cognizant Department of Defense Dependents School (DODDS) special education coordinator and/or Military Service with responsibility for Educational and Developmental Intervention Services (EDIS).

Installations. EFMP Coordinators at the medical treatment facility.

Additional information. Additional Navy EFMP information can be found in the following NAVPERSCOM publications available at each command, Fleet and Family Support Center, or Navy MTF:

- Navy Personnel Command Exceptional Family Member Program web page
- Exceptional Family Member Program Guide

Regulations

- SECNAV Instruction 1754.4B, 14 December 2005, Exceptional Family Member Program
- OPNAV 1754.2C, 22 January 2007, Exceptional Family Member Program
- BUMEDINST 1300.2A, 23 June 2006, Suitability Screening, Medical Assignment Screening and Exceptional Family Member Program (EFMP) Identification and Enrollment.

Who Is Eligible for this Program?

The Special Needs Program is available to the following members of Team Coast Guard:

- Active Duty, Retirees, and their dependents
- Civil Service employees and their dependents
- Reservists on active duty more than 180 days

Purpose of Program

The Special Needs Program is intended to ensure family and Coast Guard needs are met; assist the member with appropriate referral and resources before, during, and after relocation; and ensure mission readiness. The program works closely with assignment officers, prior to transfer, to ensure appropriate resources are available for family members in proposed areas of relocation. All active duty members who have family members with professionally diagnosed special needs are required to enroll their dependents in this program.

Definitions

The following definitions apply to the Special Needs Program:

Special Needs are long-term and professionally documented medical, educational, physical, psychological, and mental condition(s). Such conditions may include, but are not limited to:

- Vision, hearing, or speech impairment
- Learning disabilities and Attention Deficit Disorder
- Medical conditions (asthma, arthritis, heart and kidney conditions, Cystic Fibrosis, or cancer/Leukemia)
- Depression or any other mental illnesses

- Emotional disturbance
- Mental retardation
- Orthopedic handicap
- Any combination of one or more of the above

Your local Family Resource Specialist (FRS), or Family Advocacy Specialist (FAS) can advise members if their individual circumstances meet the criteria for enrollment.

Program Confidentiality

All discussions between a person using the Special Needs Program and the local Work-Life FRS or the FAS are confidential, with the exception of notification to the member's command of that member's enrollment in the program.

The FRS/FAS manage each individual member's special needs record. The information contained in that record shall not be made part of the member's service record or the civilian employee's personnel file. All information is kept confidential and access is strictly limited to the local Work-Life Supervisor, FRS, FAS, and HQ's Special Needs Program Manager.

Services and Resources Available

The following services and resources are available within the Special Needs Program:

- Assistance with enrollment in the program
- Resources and referrals
- Advocacy on behalf of families with the Coast Guard and with civilian agencies
- Assurance that appropriate resources are available in areas of proposed relocation by working closely with assignment officers and other Work-Life Staffs.

Related Program Information

- Active duty members shall not be adversely affected in their selection for promotion, schools, or assignments due to enrollment in the program
- Active duty members will be enrolled in the program until the member has separated from the service, the family member is no longer a dependent, or professional documentation has been provided verifying the

special needs condition no longer exists
- Active duty members are required to update their dependent's special needs enrollment forms (one for each family member) and professional documentation every two years or sooner if the special needs condition changes significantly
- Enrollment, resources, and assistance are also available for retirees and civilian employees

Requesting Services or Resources

These services or resources can be obtained by contacting the FRS or FAS at your Regional Work-Life Staff. Work-Life Staffs are located at Integrated Support Commands CG-wide and at the Headquarters Support Command.

Program References

The following references provide details of the Coast Guard Special Needs Program:

- **Coast Guard Special Needs Program**—COMDTINST 1754.7A
- **Management of Family Advocacy and Special Needs Cases**—COMDTINST 1754.12

Related Websites

The following websites provide information related to the Special Needs Program:

- **Air Force Crossroads (Special Needs section)**—www.afcrossroads. com/education/k12_special.cfm. Includes information on general resources; organizations; special education laws; inclusive educational programs; individualized education plans; special needs friendly colleges; ADD and ADHD; autism, Asperger's and pervasive development disorders; blind; deaf; Down syndrome and mental retardation; dyslexia; gifted; and other disabilities.
- **National Dissemination Center for Children with Disabilities (NICHCY)**—nichcy.org/index.html#about
- **PAVE**—www.washingtonpave.org/, a parent-directed organization, exists to increase independence, empowerment, and future opportunities for consumers with special needs, their families and communities, through training, information, referral, and support.

- **Special Needs Network of the Military Family Resource Center**—www.milspouse.org/Benefits/SpChild/. Site offers families with special medical and/or educational needs access to information, resources and each other. Features a "members network" that allows you to communicate with other families with special needs.
- **STOMP** (Specialized Training of Military Parents)—www.stompproject.org/default.asp. A federally funded Parent Training and Information (PTI) Center established to assist military families who have children with special education or health needs. STOMP began in 1985; it is a project of Washington PAVE, and is funded through a grant from the U.S. Department of Education.

U.S. Coast Guard Special Needs Program

The U.S. Coast Guard Special Needs Program is intended to ensure family and Coast Guard needs are met; assist the member with appropriate referral and resources before, during, and after relocation; and ensure mission readiness. The program works closely with assignment officers, prior to transfer, to ensure appropriate resources are available for family members in proposed areas of relocation. All active duty members who have family members with professionally diagnosed special needs are **required** to enroll their dependents in this program.

Enrollment

EFMP enrollment is mandatory and required immediately upon identification of a special need. The required forms for enrollment are:

- DD Form 2792, Exceptional Family Member Medical Summary for medical issues only
- DD Form 2792-1, Exceptional Family Member Special Education/Early Intervention Summary for educational issues

WHAT TO EXPECT FROM YOUR EFMP PROGRAM COORDINATOR

For military families located near an installation, there will be a special needs point of contact whose primary duties include one-on-one assistance and advocacy on behalf of special needs families. The Army and Marine Corps have EFMP Managers located in their family centers. The Navy and Air Force have EFMP/Special Needs Coordinators in their medical treatment facilities.

The program coordinator can help with enrollment and screening and give advice on the paperwork that has to be filed and presented. He or she can also advise you on your rights and responsibilities and provide information about support services available in your area. They can also help coordinate any special needs you and your family may have with you gaining installation.

The Medical Case Coordinator acts as the liaison between the program coordinator and program manager and the medical facilities.

Many installations now have a School Liaison Officer (SLO), whose role is to work with local schools in support of students from military families. They can be particularly helpful in advocating for parents of students transitioning from one school to another. The SLO should be knowledgeable about special education legal requirements and prepared to intervene on parents' behalf when they believe their child's special education needs are not being met.

OTHER CONSIDERATIONS

Respite Care and Funds

Respite care is temporary care for a disabled person for the purpose of giving the primary caregiver, usually a parent, relief from the routine of daily caregiving. Respite care may be for a few hours, so the primary caregiver can attend to personal needs, or for a few days, so the family can have a much-needed vacation. Occasional respite care helps to relieve the stress of caring for a disabled child and thus helps to prevent abuse and neglect and strengthen family stability. Services can be provided in the EFM's home, in the respite caregiver's home, or in a care facility.

TRICARE Extended Care Health Option (See Insurance)

The TRICARE Extended Care Health Option (ECHO) program has a respite care benefit. Many parents who need respite care do not qualify under ECHO, but there are other respite care options and funding sources available from both military and civilian agencies.

Eligibility for the Army's Respite Care Program is based on EFMP enrollment status, the exceptional family member's medical or educational condition, and deployment needs.

The Marine Corps EFMP Respite Care is a program that provides temporary rest periods for family members responsible for the regular care of persons with disabilities. The Marine Corps EFMP Respite Care program provides up to 40 hours of respite care monthly for EFMP enrolled families.

Respite Care may be provided by the installation CDC, FCC Home, visiting nursing service, family member, or neighbor. Interested families should contact their local installation EFMP Coordinator.

New Parent Support Program

This is a voluntary program developed to assist families expecting a child, or with a child under six years of age. A professional team of social workers and nurses provide supportive and caring services to military families through home visitation, support groups, and classes. NPSP helps families cope with the stress of parenting, deployment and reunion issues, isolation, and other issues impacting parents and children.

Counseling

Counseling or "talking therapy" involves a trained professional assisting a member in resolving problems or making a change. Counseling can be done one-on-one or as couples or groups. It can be helpful for a number of concerns such as stress symptoms, poor sleep, nervousness, tension headaches, relationship difficulties, work problems, depression, and anxiety disorders.

2

Diagnoses

DISCOVERING THAT YOUR CHILD HAS A DELAY OR DISABILITY

Learning that your child is developmentally delayed or has a disability can be a stunning blow. Many parents experience an array of feelings, frequently starting with denial and flowing into anger, fear, and guilt. It can be hard to believe that the diagnosis is true. As this new information is absorbed, anger is often present and may be directed at medical personnel or whoever provides information about the child's condition. Anger may even spill out onto family members as they try to understand what this diagnosis means. Fear stems from the unknown about what the future holds, as well as the realization that the complex job of raising a disabled child lies ahead. Many parents also experience guilt and worry that they did something to cause the disability. Sadness and disappointment are inevitable as you realize you must revise the hopes and dreams you had for your child.

You may be flooded with emotion and feel overwhelmed. However, there are constructive actions that can be taken now, and there are many sources of help, support, and reassurance available.

Reach Out

First of all, ask any questions you may have of the professional who is seeing your child. If a doctor or professional uses words you don't understand, ask them to explain. Don't be embarrassed to say, "Would you please explain that again?" A large amount of information is being absorbed and it can be very confusing. If unsure about the diagnosis, ask for a second opinion; you are entitled to one.

Some parents feel:

Denial. Often the first reaction people have to any loss is denial. When you have just learned that your child may have a disability, denial may propel you to get a second opinion. That is a good idea; doctors are imperfect.

Guilt. It is not unusual for parents to blame themselves for having done or not done something that caused their child's impairment. This can be especially difficult for mothers who may look back on their pregnancy and wonder if something they did caused their child's disability or illness.

Anger. Anger is a reasonable reaction to the loss of something precious, and you are entitled to feel angry. You might be asking, "Why me? Why my child?" Eventually, many parents use their anger to energize themselves in the struggle to get the best possible services for their child.

Sorrow. Sadness and disappointment are inevitable as you realize that the future you had envisioned for your child might never materialize. Grief is the natural reaction to loss, and if you discover that your child is especially challenged, you may need to grieve for the healthy child you had dreamed of.

Anxiety and Fear. When you learn that your child is not developing in a typical way, there is good reason to be afraid and anxious. Coping with a child who has a disability or is chronically ill can be exhausting and confusing. Worries about the future and your own ability to be a good parent are common.

Acceptance and Hope. Finally, the roller coaster ride starts to level out occasionally. Your child is still disabled or delayed, but you have a greater understanding of his or her condition and you realize that you can take good and loving care of this child. You realize that while your child may not be typical, he or she is loving and lovable.

What Can I Do?

Learn about Your Child's Condition. Search your library and the Internet for information on your child's condition. Ask your doctor any questions you have about your child's condition. Jot down questions that occur to you as you go through your day. If you don't understand something don't be embarrassed to say so.

Contact STOMP. Specialized Training of Military Parents is a valuable online resource. You will find support and advice for military parents regardless of special challenges your child may face. Join the list serve and correspond with other parents of specially challenged children at www.stompproject.org or call 1-800-5-parent.

Seek Other Parents of Children with Disabilities. Realize that you are not alone. Your Exceptional Family Member Program representative can help you find other military families who have faced similar challenges. To find the closest Family Service Center and EFMP Coordinator, go to www.militaryinstallations.dod/mil.

Seek Out Your State Parent Training Center. Every state has Parent Training Centers (PTCs). PTCs serve families with children with all disabilities, and can help you obtain appropriate educational services for your child. PTCs train parents and professionals and can help resolve problems between schools and families. To find a Parent Training Center in your state, go to www.taalliance.org.

Seek Other Parents Whose Children Have Disabilities. Contact your Exceptional Family Member Program representative at the nearest Family Support Center and ask for assistance finding families who have dealt with similar challenges.

Family Connections

Keep talking to your spouse. The more you can communicate in challenging times the greater your strength as a couple will be. You will probably not react to this new information about your child the same way, but try to explain how you feel and listen carefully as your spouse shares feelings as well. Sometimes agreement is less important than understanding. If there are other children in the home, be aware of their needs as well. If talking about the disability is too difficult at this time, ask another adult to try to establish a bond with your child so that your child has someone to talk to about his or her feelings without upsetting mom or dad.

EARLY INTERVENTION

IDEA

In 1986, Congress recognized the importance of getting early help to children with special needs and their families, so an amendment was made to the Education for All Handicapped Children Act of 1975. This ensured that children with special needs would not have to wait until they were of school age to receive services. Today, the Individuals with Disabilities Education Act (IDEA) Part C requires all fifty states and jurisdictions to have a system of early intervention for all children with disabilities from birth until they turn three. For more information about IDEA, go to www.wrightslaw.com.

What Is Early Intervention?

Every baby and child develops at a unique speed emotionally, intellectually, and physically. When children under the age of 3 are discovered to have, or be at risk of developing, a condition or special need that may affect their development, early intervention services can help the children and their families to identify and minimize these delays.

Goals of Early Intervention

Early intervention provides services with the goal of lessening the effect of any condition that may limit a child's development. It can be remedial or preventive in nature, minimizing delays or preventing their occurrence. Early intervention focuses on the child, but is most effective when the focus is on the child and the family together. Services may begin anywhere between birth and age 3; however, there are many reasons to begin as early as possible.

Why Start So Young?

There are many reasons to introduce an exceptional child to early intervention as soon as possible. The most important reason is that a child's rate of learning and development is most rapid in the preschool years. If, during these early stages of development, the teachable moments and times of greatest readiness are not taken advantage of, the same skills may take longer to learn when the child is older.

Early Intervention Strengthens Families

Early intervention is also a valuable resource for the parents and siblings of an exceptional child. The families of exceptional children may feel isolated, disappointed, frustrated, or helpless. All of these stresses may affect the whole family's well-being, as well as the child's development. Early intervention helps families to be empowered as they negotiate their way through life with a specially challenged child. It can result in parents having improved attitudes about themselves and their child as well as better information and skills for teaching their child.

Who Provides the Services?

Early intervention services are required by law and are available throughout the fifty states and U.S. territories. Each state decides which of its agencies will be in charge of early services for infants and toddlers with special needs.

Most Services Are Free

Part C of IDEA requires that the evaluation or assessments, the development of an Individual Family Service Plan (IFSP), and the service coordination be provided free of charge to eligible children and their families. Other services may also be provided at no cost to families, although some fees may be assessed on a sliding scale depending on the income of the child's family. However, the law also states that no family shall be denied services because they cannot afford them. If you have problems with cost or availability of services, contact your service coordinator or your health benefits advisor. Early intervention may be paid for under your TRICARE option, your private insurance, or Medicaid. Each child's family has the final say on what services they will accept, and they may reject services they don't want to pay for.

The Department of Defense also has an early intervention program to meet the needs of children who reside on military bases with DoD schools but are too young to attend. All DoD Early Intervention Services are provided at no charge.

Referrals and Service Coordinators

Referrals for Early Intervention Services are usually made by a child's parents or physician, but they can be made by anyone on behalf of a family. Once a child has been referred for EIS, a service coordinator will be assigned to assist the family by gathering information from the family, arranging for appropriate assessments and evaluations, and eventually creating an Individual Family Service Plan. Your service coordinator will be your contact as evaluations are conducted and meetings are scheduled to discuss the results and will help with assessing and coordinating recommended services.

The Evaluation Process

Within 45 calendar days of the referral, an evaluation must be completed and a service plan put in place if the child is found to be eligible for early intervention. The evaluation will determine whether or not a child needs early intervention services. It consists of a general developmental assessment of the child's abilities, including the following:

A parent interview to voice concerns about a child's delay(s).
A review of the child's medical history.
Assessments by specialists in the areas of concern

The following areas will be assessed:

Physical development. The ability to see, to hear, and to move with purpose or coordination.

Language and speech development. The ability to talk, to understand language, and to express needs.

Social and emotional development. The ability of a child with typical intelligence to build satisfactory relationships and respond appropriately under normal circumstances.

Adaptive development. The ability to eat, to dress, to toilet, and to perform other self-help skills.

Cognitive development. The ability to think and to learn; a measurement of intellectual functioning which is related to the child's ability to think, to speak, to read, to write, or to do mathematical calculations.

To minimize anxiety during the assessment process, do not allow your child to be separated from you. The anxiety of separation may cause a child to do poorly. Make sure the child is comfortable with the professional doing the assessment. This may take time and require more than one session. The goal is a fair assessment of the child's abilities and weaknesses.

Discussing Your Child's Special Challenges

Many parents have mixed feelings about discussing their child's area of weakness. It may feel unloving or disloyal to call attention to the child's delays. However, spelling out concerns and noticing the areas of weakness is your responsibility as your child's advocate. Your child will benefit when, because of your shared observations, needed services are made available. Being very honest is a loving choice.

Who Is Eligible?

Babies and children may be eligible for services until they turn 3 if they meet the following criteria:

The child has a diagnosed physical or mental condition which is likely to result in a delay of development.

The child has a developmental delay in one or more of the following areas: cognitive (intellect), physical development (to include vision and hearing), social or emotional development, self-help or adaptive skills.

The child is considered to be at high risk of developing substantial delays if early intervention is not provided.

The Eligibility Meeting

After assessments have been completed, an eligibility meeting will be held. The evaluations and observations of the child will be compared with the eligibility criteria listed above to determine whether the child qualifies for services. It is at this meeting that a child will or will not be found eligible for services.

Preparing for the Eligibility Meeting

To prepare for this meeting, gather and write down your own information about your child's growth and development and be prepared to share this with the team. You may want to make a small poster about your child to help the team to better know your child and to remember that he or she is unique and much loved. It is helpful to bring a family member or friend with you. Often you will have been given the results of the screening of your child. You may be pleasantly surprised, or dismayed, by the findings. Don't rush through these meetings. Ask questions of the professionals in the room about your child's ability levels or services you believe might be a help to your child or your family. Remember that formal testing is just one component of your child's assessment. Your observations and experiences with your child are an important component of the assessment. Don't give up if the assessment team does not place the same importance on an observation as you do. Talk it over with them so that you are able to understand their point of view, and they understand yours.

A Parent's Perspective

It may feel uncomfortable explaining to a stranger that something is not quite right about your child. It may be tempting to minimize your child's delay because you are so proud of the gains your child has made and because you love your child so profoundly. Keep in mind that in order for your child to qualify for appropriate services there must be a clear and accurate picture of your child's development.

Individual Family Support Plans

If a child is found eligible for Early Intervention Services, parents and members of their support team will gather again to write an Individual Family Support Plan (IFSP). This plan will identify what the child's current developmental levels are, what services will be provided to advance those levels, and what goals parents would like to see their child reach. Armed with this information, you will be able to specify the direction you would like to see your child move in and to identify milestones along the way. The IFSP will contain valuable information about your child's strengths, needs, likes, and dislikes. This information, combined with results from assessments and medical information from your child's doctor, will provide a thorough description of your child's special needs and goals.

Families will revisit this document with their child's service coordinator regularly to assess how goals are being met and to revise or update the steps being taken to assist their child.

The IFSP will include the following components:

Information about your child's current development
Information about family resources, priorities, and concerns
Goals of the plan
Detailed description of services needed to help your child reach goals
Statement about the natural environment where the services will be provided
Start date for services and the expected duration
Name of the service coordinator who will help obtain the services identified
Transition plan for your child

The IFSP Meeting

The guiding principal of the IFSP is that the family is a child's greatest resource and that a baby's needs are closely tied to the needs of the family. The best way to support children and meet their needs is to support and build on the individual strengths of their family. So the IFSP is a whole-family plan with the parents as the most important part of the IFSP team.

Preparing for Your IFSP Meeting

Sitting down with a room full of professionals to discuss challenges and opportunities for your child can be difficult and emotionally draining. However, you are the leading expert on your child, and your input is crucial to the quality of the IFSP. To ensure that you remember to discuss all your hopes and concerns, it is helpful to write down observations and areas of concern in the days before the meeting. If IFSP meetings are emotionally difficult and no family member is available to attend with you, ask a friend who is familiar with your child to accompany you. This person can offer moral support as well as another view point on the situation. The IFSP will be reviewed at regular intervals to monitor your child's progress and adjust goals accordingly.

Types of Services

The IFSP will define what type of intervention will best benefit your child and your family. The services that are required to be made available to eligible families include the following:

Assistive Technology. Devices or services that allow or improve independence in daily activities (e.g., a curved handle on a spoon for easier self-feeding or a wheel chair).

Audiology. Therapy for individuals with hearing loss.

Family Training. May be counseling to help family understand the special needs of their child and how to best support the child's development.

Medical Services. For birth to age 3 for diagnostic or evaluation purposes only.

Nursing Services. May assess health status of your child or administer treatments prescribed by a physician.

Nutrition Services. Address the nutritional needs of your child and may include identifying feeding skills or problems, food habits, or preferences.

Occupational Therapy. Activities designed to improve fine motor skills (e.g., finger, hand, or arm movements).

Physical Therapy. Activities designed to improve gross motor skills (e.g., leg, back, or whole body movements).

Psychological Services. Administering and interpreting psychological tests and information about a child's behavior; may include counseling, parent training, and education programs.

Respite Care. Trained caregivers who will take care of your child, giving you a little time off.

Service Coordination. Bringing together the people, information, and resources that your child and family may need.

Specialized Instruction. Programs or services specially designed to meet the needs of children with special needs.

Speech and Language Services. Activities and materials designed to improve your child's ability to express thoughts and information.

Transportation. Providing for the travel necessary to enable a child and family to receive early intervention services.

Vision Services. Identification of, and services for, children with visual disorders or delays.

Making the Most of Available Services

As a parent, it is very important to watch how your child is taught and encouraged while receiving services. By modeling this behavior at home, you
are reinforcing the lessons and increasing the speed at which your child will
master the new skills being addressed. Every session, whether at home or at a
center, offers a chance for the service provider and the family to share information about the child. A child's parents know the child best and can share
daily observations. The service provider can offer ideas on how to help the
child in the home environment. A cooperative partnership between the family, the service coordinator, the teachers, and the service provider will benefit
the child profoundly.

Your Role as Advocate

When a parent first realizes that a child may face more challenges than his or her
peers, the reaction can be an emotional one. Over time, the family accepts that
it has different circumstances than most. The realization that children will need
specific services to mitigate these delays turns many parents into advocates.

Parents are natural advocates for their children. They are their child's first
teachers, they know their child better than anyone else, and they have their
child's best interests at heart. Children need their parents to play an active
role in planning their education. The law gives parents the power to make
educational decisions for their child. How can this power be best used to
benefit the child?

Your Rights

Parents have certain rights under the Individuals with Disabilities Act. They
have the right to do the following:

Choose whether or not to have a child evaluated and if so, to have it done
in a timely manner.
Go through the early intervention process in their own language.
Receive full copies of all evaluation results and notices regarding each
aspect of the program.
Refuse any specific service without losing the right to other services.
Bring or consult an advocate or attorney to any meeting or stage of the process.
Keep all information regarding the family confidential.
Examine and correct all records regarding the child and family.
Withhold or withdraw consent at any stage of the process.

Be told of any possible changes in the child's evaluation or services before any are made.

Be involved in all stages of early intervention.

Not to participate in the Early Intervention Program.

The role as a parent is vital, for parents are the most important people in their child's life and they know their child best. Make sure that early intervention services are doing what is best for your child.

To ensure this, be ready to organize and keep track of all the paperwork throughout the early intervention process. Learn about assistive technology so you will be informed enough to ask for devices that might aid your child. Be aware of your rights and those of your family and be an active participant in all stages of early intervention.

CHALLENGES AND SUPPORT

Sometimes, even though parents may suspect their child has a delay, they hesitate to ask for help, perhaps hoping that the child will catch up to his or her peers without additional help. If you are hesitating, consider that there is nothing to lose by asking to have your child screened. Either necessary help will be offered, or you will receive reassuring answers to your questions.

Challenges

Learning how to find appropriate services for your child can be difficult, and military families must also deal with the complication of relocating and starting the process again. It is very important to carry the documentation of your child's early intervention program with you to your new home. Once in the new location, seek early intervention services quickly, as there may be a waiting list or other delays in services. Call the National Dissemination Center for Children with Disabilities (NICHCY) at 1-800-695-0285 to find who provides early intervention in your area.

Although all states have early intervention services, all programs are not equal and a child may not be eligible for the same services at the new location. Also, you may need to demonstrate residency before you can apply for services.

Support

Members of the military have many groups and agencies to turn to for help with their exceptional children. Please take advantage of the many resources that have been put in place. Remember that you are not alone and there are knowl-edgeable people ready and waiting to help. Being the caretakers of a child with special needs can be physically exhausting as well as emotionally draining. By finding people to talk to about your life, your child, and your unique stresses, you will be helping yourself as well as your child. Caretakers need care too. If you think you might benefit from counseling, contact your family service center at www.militaryinstallations.dod.mil or Military OneSource at www.militaryonesource.com or call 1-800-342-9647. Help is close by.

FOR MORE INFORMATION

Obtain the other modules of the Parent Tool Kit at www.militaryhomefront.dod.mil/efm or from your EFMP coordinator.

 Module Two, *Special Education*
 Module Three, *Health Benefits*
 Module Four, *Families in Transition*
 Module Five, *Advocating for Your Child*
 Module Six, *Resources and Support*

 For parents of babies and toddlers who are newly diagnosed with a devel-opmental delay or disability, the following resources are especially helpful.

STOMP

Specialized Training of Military Parents (STOMP) is a national organization dedicated to educating and training military parents of children who have special education or health-care needs. STOMP assists military families by providing information, support, and advice. STOMP can also connect you to other military families with exceptional children. Visit the STOMP website and consider joining their list serve at www.stompproject.org.

Parent Training Centers

Another resource is your state's Parent Training Center. Each state has a minimum of one Parent Training Center that is designed to serve families of children and young adults from birth to age 22 with all disabilities. Centers may provide information, training, referrals, and advocacy services to help parents obtain the needed resources within their communities. To locate the Parent Training Center within your state, visit www.taalliance.org.

NICHCY

The National Dissemination Center for Children with Disabilities (NICHCY) offers a wealth of information in both English and Spanish. To learn more about early intervention for infant and toddlers and specific disabilities, visit their website at www.nichcy.org.

Wrightslaw

Parents, advocates, educators, and attorneys utilize Wrightslaw for accurate, up-to-date information about special education law and advocacy for children with disabilities. You will find articles, cases, newsletters, and resources about the Individual with Disabilities Education Act (IDEA) and other legal issues at www.wrightslaw.com.

DISEASES, DISORDERS, AND SYNDROMES

- *Acid Maltase*
  - The Acid Maltase Deficiency Association (AMDA)—The Acid Maltase Deficiency Association, AMDA, was formed to assist in funding research and to promote public awareness of Acid Maltase Deficiency, also known as Pompe's Disease.
  - Making Headway Foundation, Inc.—Making Headway is a support program for families of children with brain and spinal cord tumors and other catastrophic neurological illnesses. The programs and support services cover care before surgery, during the hospital stay, and after the child returns home.
- *Acidemia, Organic*
  - Organic Acidemia Association—The Organic Acidemia Association is a voluntary not-for-profit self-help organization dedicated to providing information and support to families of children with inborn errors of metabolism. The Organic Acidemia Association provides information to affected families and health-care professionals across the country and internationally.
- *Acoustic Neuroma*
  - The Acoustic Neuroma Association—The Acoustic Neuroma Association provides information and support to patients who have been diagnosed with or experienced an acoustic neuroma or other benign problem affecting the cranial nerves.

- *Adrenal Disorders*
  - o National Adrenal Diseases Foundation—The National Adrenal Diseases Foundation is a nonprofit organization dedicated to providing support, information, and education to individuals having Addison's disease as well as other diseases of the adrenal glands.
- *Agenesis of the Corpus Callosum*
  - o National Organization of Disorders of the Corpus Callosum (NODCC)—NODCC's mission is to enhance the quality of life of individuals with agenesis of the corpus callosum and other disorders of the corpus callosum by gathering and disseminating information regarding these conditions.
- *Aicardi Syndrome*
  - o Aicardi Syndrome—Provides information and comfort to families and friends of girls diagnosed with Aicardi Syndrome.
- *Albinism Hypopigmentation*
  - o NOAH—NOAH is a U.S.-based nonprofit, tax-exempt organization that offers information and support to people with albinism, their families, and the professionals who work with them.
- *Alopecia Areata*
  - o National Alopecia Areata Foundation—The mission of the National Alopecia Areata Foundation (NAAF) is to support research to find a cure or acceptable treatment for alopecia areata, to support those with the disease, and to educate the public about alopecia areata.
- *Alpha-1-Antitrypsin (AAT) Deficiency*
  - o ALPHA-1 National Association—Clearinghouse of information, support, and education for people bearing Alpha-1 Antitrypsin Deficiency.
- *Alstrom Syndrome*
  - o Alstrom Syndrome Newsletter—To provide support, information, and coordination worldwide to families and professionals in order to treat and cure Alstrom Syndrome. Can lend support to patients, families, and physicians confronting the difficulties posed by Alstrom Syndrome.
- *Anathalmia*
  - o International Children's Network—ican (International Children's Anophthalmia Network) is a parent support group for families with a child with anophthalmia or microphthalmia.
- *Angelman Syndrome*
  - o Angelman Syndrome Foundation—Information about ASF.
- *Anophthalmia*
- International Children's Anophthalmia Network (ican)—A support group for individuals with anophthalmia, micropthalmia, and coloboma, and their families.

- *Anorectal Malformations*
  o Pull-Thru Network—The Pull-thru Network was organized as a chapter of the United Ostomy Association by a group of families whose children were born with an anorectal malformation. The PTN is dedicated to the support and information needs of the families of children born with imperforate anus, cloaca, cloaca exstrophy, bladder exstrophy, VATER Syndrome, Hirschsprung's Disease, and other related birth anomalies.
- *Anorexia Nervosa*
  o National Eating Disorder Association—The National Eating Disorders Association (NEDA) is a not-for-profit organization in the United States working to prevent eating disorders and provide treatment referrals to those suffering from anorexia, bulimia, and binge eating disorder and those concerned with body image and weight issues.
- *Aphasia*
  o National Aphasia Association (NAA)—NAA is a nonprofit organization that promotes public education, research, rehabilitation, and support services to assist people with aphasia and their families.
- *Aplastic Anemia*
  o Aplastic Anemia and MDS International Foundation, Inc.—The Aplastic Anemia and MDS International Foundation is the largest patient advocate and support organization for bone marrow diseases, providing life-saving hope, knowledge, and support to hundreds of thousands of patients and their families.
- *Apraxia*
  o C.H.E.R.A.B. Foundation, Inc.—Provides communication help, education, and research.
  o The Childhood Apraxia of Speech Association—A 501(c)(3) nonprofit publicly funded charity whose mission is to strengthen the support systems in the lives of children with apraxia so that each child is afforded their best opportunity to develop speech.
- *Arnold Chiari Malformation*
  o National Institute of Neurological Disorders and Stroke (NINDS)— The mission of NINDS is to reduce the burden of neurological disease—a burden borne by every age group, by every segment of society, by people all over the world.
- *Arthritis*
  o Arthritis Foundation—Information about arthritis.
  o National Institute of Arthritis and Musculoskeletal and Skin Diseases Information Clearinghouse (NIAMS)—supports research into the causes, treatment, and prevention of arthritis and musculoskeletal and

skin diseases; trains basic and clinical scientists to carry out this research and disseminates information on research progress in these diseases.

- *Asthma and Allergy*
  - o Allergy and Asthma Network; Mothers of Asthmatics (AANMA)— AANMA is a national nonprofit network of families whose desire is to overcome, not cope with, allergies and asthma.
  - o Asthma and Allergy Foundation of America—Helps with education, advocacy, research, publications, chapters, and support groups. Get quick facts about asthma, allergies (including food allergies) and more!
- *Ataxia*
  - o Ataxia—The National Ataxia Foundation is a nonprofit organization with the primary mission of encouraging and supporting research into Hereditary Ataxia, a group of neurological disorders that are chronic and progressive conditions affecting coordination.
- *Ataxia Telangiectasia*
  - o A-T Children's Project—A-T Children's Project was formed to raise funds through events and contributions from corporations, foundations and friends. These funds are then used to accelerate first-rate, international scientific research aimed at finding a cure and improving the lives of all children with Ataxia Telangiectasia.
- *Attention Deficit Disorder (ADD)*
  - o Children and Adults with ADD (CHADD)—CHADD has more than 16,000 members in 200 local chapters throughout the United States. Chapters offer support for individuals, parents, teachers, professionals, and others.
  - o National Attention Deficit Disorder Association—The mission of ADDA is to provide information, resources, and networking to adults with AD/HD and to the professionals who work with them.
- *Autism*
  - o Autism in the Criminal Justice System—This video illustrates verbal and nonverbal communications difficulties experienced by persons with autism who may become victims, witnesses, or offenders in the criminal justice system, and offers advice and information for criminal justice professionals who may interact with them. The video features persons with autism, criminal justice professionals and autism professionals through vignette and interviews and was produced to enhance communications and facilitate understanding of autism in the criminal justice system.
  - o Autism National Committee—Founded in 1990 to protect and advance the human rights and civil rights of all persons with autism, Pervasive Developmental Disorder, and related differences of communication and behavior.

o Autism—NIH Study—This monograph by the National Institutes of Health (NIH) describes how scientists have come one step closer to determining the genetic basis for autism. The researchers have identified regions of four chromosomes that appear to be linked with the disorder.

o Autism Society of America—The mission of the Autism Society of America is to promote lifelong access and opportunity for all individuals within the autism spectrum, and their families, to be fully participating, included members of their community. Education, advocacy at state and federal levels, active public awareness, and the promotion of research form the cornerstones of ASA's efforts to carry forth its mission.

o Autism Services North—A TRICARE-approved Applied Behavior Analysis (ABA) provider serving military families in TRICARE's North, West, and South regions.

o Cleveland Clinic Children's Hospital Center for Autism—Located in Cleveland, Ohio, the Center for Autism offers behavioral health services, diagnostic services, workshops, and more.

o Educating Children with Autism—National Academy of Education report on educating children with autism.

o Kennedy Krieger Institute: Center for Autism and Related Disorders—Kennedy Krieger's clinical programs offer an interdisciplinary approach in treatment tailored to the individual needs of each child. Services include over forty outpatient clinics; neurobehavioral, rehabilitation, and pediatric feeding disorders inpatient units; plus several home and community programs providing services to assist families.

o Operation Autism: A Resource Guide for Military Families—Operation Autism directly supports U.S. military families touched by autism and autism spectrum disorders. It serves as an introduction to autism, a guide for the life journey with autism, and a ready reference for available resources, services, and support. Also available is *A Guide for Military Families,* the purpose of which is to give military families touched by autism the tools and access to information they need to navigate their unique life journeys.

o Treatment and Education of Autistic and Communication Related Handicapped Children (TEACCH)—"Evidence-based service, training, and research program for individuals of all ages and skill levels with autism spectrum disorders" (www.teacch.com).

o The Dan Marino Foundation—The mission of the Dan Marino Foundation is to support integrated treatment programs for children with chronic illnesses and developmental disabilities, so they can lead healthier and happier lives.

o The Doug Flutie Jr. Foundation for Autism, Inc.—The foundation's mission is to aid financially disadvantaged families who need assistance in caring for their children with autism; to fund education and research into the causes and consequences of childhood autism; and to serve as a clearinghouse and communications center for new programs and services developed for individuals with autism.

o Yale Program for Autism, Prader-Willi Syndrome, and Williams Syndrome—The Yale Developmental Disabilities Clinic offers comprehensive, multidisciplinary evaluations for children with social disabilities, usually focusing on the issues of diagnosis and intervention.

- *Autoimmune Disorders*
  o Autoimmune Disorders—Patient information on more than 56 autoimmune related diseases.
- *Balance and Dizziness Disorders*
  o EAR Foundation—The Ear Foundation website has been designed to be a resource to provide information to people who suffer from impaired hearing as well as for the people who live and work with these individuals.
- *Barth Syndrome*
  o The Barth Syndrome Foundation, Inc.—The foundation's mission is to guide the search for a cure, to educate and support physicians, and to create a caring community for affected families.
- *Batten Disease*
  o Batten Disease Support and Research Association—An international support and research networking organization for families of children and young adults with an inherited neurological degenerative disorder known as Batten Disease.
- *Beckwith-Wiedemann Syndrome*
  o Beckwith-Wiedemann Support Network (BWSN)—The BWSN is a nonprofit organization created for parents, professionals, and others interested in the Beckwith-Wiedemann Syndrome. (This website has a parent forum.)
- *Bone and Marrow Transplant*
  o Blood and Marrow Transplant Information Network—A not-for-profit organization dedicated exclusively to serving the needs of persons facing a bone marrow, blood stem cell, or umbilical cord blood transplant.
- *Brain Injury*
  o Brain Injury Association of America—By acting as a clearinghouse of community service information and resources, participating in legislative advocacy, facilitating prevention awareness, hosting educational programs, and encouraging research, the Brain Injury Association of

America and its affiliates reach the millions of individuals living with the "silent epidemic" of brain injury.

- **Brain Tumor**
  - o The Brain Tumor Society—This society exists to find a cure for brain tumors. It strives to improve the quality of life of brain tumor patients and their families. It disseminates educational information and provides access to psychosocial support. It raises funds to advance carefully selected scientific research projects, improve clinical care, and find a cure.
  - o Children's Brain Tumor Foundation—was founded by families, friends, and physicians of children with brain tumors. The foundation's mission is to raise funds for scientific research and heighten public awareness of this most devastating disease and to improve prognosis and quality of life for those that are affected.
- **Burns**
  - o Phoenix Society for Burn Survivors—For over 25 years, the Phoenix Society for Burn Survivors, Inc., has been connecting burn survivors, their loved ones, and burn care professionals with valuable resources.
- **Cancer**
  - o American Cancer Society—A nationwide community-based voluntary health organization dedicated to eliminating cancer as a major health problem by preventing cancer, saving lives, and diminishing suffering from cancer, through research, education, advocacy, and service.
  - o Candlelighters Childhood Cancer Foundation—This foundation is committed to their mission of providing support, education, and advocacy for children and adolescents with cancer, survivors of childhood/adolescent cancer, their families, and the professionals who care for them.
  - o National Childhood Cancer Foundation (CureSearch)—CureSearch unites the world's largest childhood cancer research organization, the Children's Oncology Group, and the National Childhood Cancer Foundation through their shared mission to cure childhood cancer.
- **Celiac Disease**
  - o Celiac Disease Foundation (CDF)—CDF provides support, information, and assistance to people affected by Celiac Disease/Dermatitis Herpetiformis (CD/DH).
  - o Celiac Sprue Association—A national education organization that provides information and referral services for persons with the conditions of nontropical sprue (celiac disease) and dermatitis herpetiformis and for parents of celiac children.
- **Cerebral Palsy**
  - o Kennedy Krieger Institute Phelps Center for Cerebral Palsy and Neurodevelopmental Medicine

o United Cerebral Palsy Association—Their mission is to advance the independence, productivity, and full citizenship of people with cerebral palsy and other disabilities, through their commitment to the principles of independence, inclusion, and self-determination.

- *Charcot-Marie-Tooth Disease*
  o Charcot-Marie-Tooth Association—This website provides a list of support groups and publications about Charcot-Marie-Tooth Disease.
- *Charge Syndrome*
  o Velo-Cardio-Facial Syndrome; VACTERL Association; Charge Syndrome Foundation, Inc.—The mission of the CHARGE Syndrome Foundation is to provide support to individuals with CHARGE syndrome and their families; to gather, develop, maintain, and distribute information about CHARGE syndrome; and to promote awareness and research regarding its identification, cause, and management.
- *Chronic Fatigue Syndrome*
  o CFIDS Association of America—The CFIDS Association of America is the nation's leading charitable organization dedicated to conquering chronic fatigue and immune dysfunction syndrome (CFIDS), also known as chronic fatigue syndrome (CFS). The association plays a catalytic role in accelerating the pace of CFIDS research, achieving public policy victories for people with CFIDS, and focusing mainstream attention on this serious public health concern.
- *Cleft Palate*
  o Smiles—SMILES is a group of dedicated families who have developed a first-hand understanding of the needs of children with cleft lip, cleft palate, and craniofacial deformities. Through our personal sensitivity, energy, knowledge, and love we are dedicated to improve the lives of these children in our country and around the world.
  o Cleft Palate Foundation—A nonprofit organization dedicated to optimizing the quality of life for individuals affected by facial birth defects.
- *Coffin-Lowry Syndrome*
  o Coffin-Lowry Syndrome Foundation—Provides a clearinghouse for information on Coffin-Lowry Syndrome (CLS), and to provide families affected by Coffin-Lowry syndrome a general forum in which to exchange information, ideas, and advice.
- *Connective Tissue Disorders*
  o National Marfan Foundation—This foundation was founded in 1981 by people who have the Marfan syndrome and their families. It is a voluntary organization that has three objectives: To disseminate accurate and timely information about this condition to patients, family

members, and the health-care community; provide a network of communications for patients and relatives to share experiences, support one another, and improve their medical care; and, support and foster research.

- *Cooley's Anemia and Thalassemia*
  - o Cooley's Anemia Foundation—Information for patients and their families, medical personnel, donors, foundation volunteers, and anyone interested in learning about Cooley's Anemia and other forms of the genetic blood disorder, thalassemia.
- *Cornelia de Lange Syndrome*
  - o The Cornelia de Lange Syndrome Foundation—A family support organization that exists to ensure the early and accurate diagnosis of CdLS, promote research into the causes and manifestations of the syndrome, and help people with a diagnosis of CdLS, and others with similar characteristics, make informed decisions throughout their lifetime.
- *Craniofacial Disorders*
  - o Children's Craniofacial Association—Dedicated to improving the quality of life for people with facial differences and their families. Nationally and internationally, CCA addresses the medical, financial, psychosocial, emotional, and educational concerns relating to craniofacial conditions. CCA's mission is to empower and give hope to facially disfigured children and their families.
  - o FACES—The National Craniofacial Association—FACES is dedicated to assisting children and adults who have craniofacial disorders resulting from disease, accident, or birth.
  - o Forward Face: Helping Children with Craniofacial Conditions—Forward Face's mission is to help children with craniofacial conditions, and their families, find immediate support that helps empower them to successfully manage the craniofacial condition. Forward Face provides comprehensive services: educational support, advocacy, networking, community organizing, and other forms of assistance, when necessary.
  - o The National Foundation for Facial Reconstruction (NFFR)—A 501 (c)(3) nonprofit organization to enable patients with facial deformities to lead productive, fulfilling lives.
- *Cri Du Chat Syndrome*
  - o 5p- Society—This society's mission is to facilitate communication among families who have a child with 5p- Syndrome, to spread awareness and education of this syndrome to families and service providers.

- **Crohn's Disease and Colitis**
  - o The Crohn's and Colitis Foundation of America (CCFA)—A non-profit, volunteer-driven organization dedicated to finding the cure for Crohn's disease and ulcerative colitis.
- **Cyclic Vomiting Syndrome**
  - o Cyclic Vomiting Syndrome Association—A volunteer organization serving the needs of CVS patients worldwide, their families, and the growing medical community studying CVS.
- **Cystic Fibrosis**
  - o Cystic Fibrosis Foundation—The mission of the Cystic Fibrosis Foundation is to assure the development of the means to cure and control cystic fibrosis and to improve the quality of life for those with the disease.
- **Cystinosis**
  - o Cystinosis Research Network—A volunteer, nonprofit organization dedicated to supporting and advocating research, providing family assistance, and educating the public and medical communities about cystinosis.
- **Cystinuria**
  - o Cystinuria Support Network—The Cystinuria Support Network has been developed to provide a resource for putting individuals in touch with each other for support and practical advice.
- **Deaf-Blind**
  - o American Association for the Deaf-Blind—Their mission is to enable deaf-blind persons to achieve their maximum potential through increased independence, productivity, and integration into the community.
  - o National Family Association for Deaf-Blind (NFADB)—A nonprofit, volunteer-based family association whose philosophy is that individuals who are deaf-blind are valued members of society and are entitled to the same opportunities and choices as other members of the community.
  - o The National Clearinghouse on Children who are Deaf-Blind—DB-LINK's goal is to help parents, teachers, and others by providing them with information to foster the skills, strategies, and confidence necessary to nurture and empower deaf-blind children. DB-LINK is a federally funded service that identifies, coordinates, and disseminates, at no cost, information related to children and youth from birth through 21 years of age.
- **Diabetes**
  - o American Diabetes Association—The American Diabetes Association mission is to prevent and cure diabetes and to improve the lives of all people affected by diabetes. To fulfill this mission, the American Diabetes Association funds research, publishes scientific findings, and

provides information and other services to people with diabetes, their families, health-care professionals and the public. The association is also actively involved in advocating for scientific research and for the rights of people with diabetes.

o The Juvenile Diabetes Research Foundation International—Their mission is to find a cure for diabetes and its complications through research.

• *Down Syndrome*

o Association for Children with Down Syndrome (ACDS)—ACDS is dedicated to providing lifetime resources of exceptional quality, innovation, and inclusion for individuals with Down syndrome and other developmental disabilities and their families.

o National Down Syndrome Society—The most comprehensive online resource for information about Down syndrome.

o National Down Syndrome Congress—The mission of the NDSC is to provide information, advocacy, and support concerning all aspects of life for individuals with Down syndrome.

• *Dwarfism*

o Billy Barty Foundation—The Billy Barty Foundation's mission is to guarantee an acceptable and improved quality of life for Little People through education, employment, accessibility, and athletic programs.

• *Dysautonomia*

o The National Dysautonomia Research Foundation—A nonprofit foundation established to help those who are afflicted with any of the various forms of dysautonomia.

• *Dyslexia*

o Dyslexia Research Institute, Inc.—This organization's goal has been to change the perception of learning differences, specifically in the area of dyslexia and attention deficit disorders (ADD). With proper recognition and intervention, dyslexics and individuals with ADD become successful individuals using their talents and skills to enrich our society.

o The International Dyslexia Association (IDA)—A nonprofit organization dedicated to helping individuals with dyslexia, their families, and the communities that support them.

• *Dystonia*

o Dystonia Medical Research Foundation—Their goal is to advance research for more treatments and ultimately a cure; to promote awareness and education; and to support the needs and well-being of affected individuals and families.

• *Ectodermal Dysplasias*

o The National Foundation for Ectodermal Dysplasias (NFED)—Committed to assisting people with ectodermal dysplasia to live not only normal lifespans, but nearly normal lifestyles.

- **Ehlers-Danlos Syndrome**
  o Ehlers-Danlos National Foundation—Provides emotional support and the latest information to those affected by Ehlers-Danlos syndrome.
- **Epidermolysis Bullosa Dystrophic**
  o Dystrophic Epidermolysis Bullosa Research Association of America (DebRA)—A national nonprofit organization dedicated to both promoting research to find new treatments and a cure for Epidermolysis Bullosa and providing information and support for people with EB and their families.
- **Epilepsy**
  o The American Epilepsy Society—Promotes research and education for professionals dedicated to the prevention, treatment, and cure of epilepsy.
- **Essential Tremor**
  o International Essential Tremor Foundation (IETF)—IETF was created to provide information, services, and support to individuals and families affected by essential tremor (ET). The organization encourages and promotes research in an effort to determine the causes, treatment, and ultimately the cure for ET.
- **Exostoses**
  o The MHE Coalition—The MHE Coalition was formed to provide support and information to people living with Multiple Hereditary Exostoses (MHE) and to reach out to MHE-affected individuals and families throughout the world. This organization is dedicated to promoting and encouraging research to find the causes, treatments, and ultimately the cure for this rare bone disease.
- **Facio-Scapulo-Humeral Muscular Dystrophy**
  o FSH Society, Inc.—Addresses issues and needs related to FacioScapuloHumeral Muscular Dystrophy.
- **Fatty Oxidation Disorder**
  o FOD Family Support Group—Intended to be used as a resource for families, friends, doctors, researchers, and others who would like to support, educate, and provide a forum for the sharing of ideas and concerns for those whose lives have been touched by a fatty oxidation disorder.
- **Fetal Alcohol Syndrome**
  o Family Empowerment Network (FEN)—A national organization serving families affected by Fetal Alcohol Syndrome and Fetal Alcohol Effects as well as the professionals involved in their lives.

o National Organization on Fetal Alcohol Syndrome—Dedicated to eliminating birth defects caused by alcohol consumption during pregnancy and improving the quality of life for those individuals and families affected.

o The Fetal Alcohol Syndrome Family Resource Institute—The mission of FAS is to identify, understand, and care for individuals disabled by prenatal alcohol exposure and their families, and to prevent future generations from having to live with this disability.

o University of Washington's Fetal Alcohol and Drug Unit—The Fetal Alcohol and Drug Unit is a research unit dedicated to the prevention, intervention, and treatment of Fetal Alcohol Syndrome (FAS) and Fetal Alcohol Effects (FAE). They also provide information on their research projects and findings, have a list of support groups worldwide, list international FAS/FAE conferences as they come up, and provide many other national and international resources. The Fetal Alcohol and Drug Unit is also the home of the Fetal Alcohol Syndrome/Effects Legal Issues Resource Center.

- *Fragile X Syndrome*
  o FRAXA Research Foundation—FRAXA's mission is to accelerate progress toward effective treatments and ultimately a cure for Fragile X, by directly funding the most promising research. FRAXA also supports families affected by Fragile X and raises awareness of this important but virtually unknown disease.
  o National Fragile X Foundation—Provides support and education and raises awareness about Fragile X Syndrome.
- *Galactosemia*
  o Parents of Galactosemic Children, Inc. (PGC)—A national, nonprofit, volunteer organization whose mission is to provide information, support, and networking opportunities to families affected by galactosemia.
- *Gastrointestinal Disorders*
  o The Oley Foundation—A national, independent, nonprofit organization that provides up-to-date information, outreach services, conference activities, and emotional support for homePEN consumers, their families, caregivers, and professionals.
- *Gastrointestinal Reflux*
  o Pediatric Adolescent Gastroesophageal Reflux Association, Inc. (PAGER)—A 501(c)(3) nonprofit membership organization that provides information and support to parents, patients, and doctors about Gastroesophageal Reflux (GER). Information is available for adults.

- *Gaucher Disease*
  - o National Gaucher Foundation (NGF)—Dedicated to supporting and promoting research into the causes of, and a cure for Gaucher Disease. The mission of the NGF is to find a cure for Gaucher Disease by funding vital research programs, to meet the ever-increasing needs of patients and families, as well as to promote community/physician awareness and educational programs. The NGF offers a variety of services and programs including regional chapter meetings, patient support groups, international conferences, as well as the CARE Program and the Care+Plus Program, which provide critical financial assistance to individuals with Gaucher Disease.
- *Genetic Disorders*
  - o Genetic Alliance—An international coalition of individuals, professionals, and genetic support organizations that are working together to promote healthy lives for everyone impacted by genetics.
  - o The MAGIC Foundation—A national nonprofit organization created to provide support services for the families of children afflicted with a wide variety of chronic and/or critical disorders, syndromes, and diseases that affect a child's growth.
  - o Velo-Cardio-Facial Syndrome Educational Foundation Inc.—The Foundation is an international not-for-profit organization dedicated to providing support and information to individuals who are affected by this syndrome, their families, physicians and other practitioners.
- *Glaucoma*
  - o Glaucoma Research Foundation—A national nonprofit organization dedicated to protecting the sight and independence of people with glaucoma through research and education, with the ultimate goal of curing glaucoma. GRF funds leading-edge research around the world, seeking new and better treatments for glaucoma in addition to a cure for this devastating disease, the leading cause of preventable blindness in America.
- *Gluten Intolerance*
  - o Gluten Intolerance Group of North America—This group's mission is to increase awareness by providing current, accurate, information and education, as well as support, to persons with gluten intolerance diseases, such as celiac disease and dermatitis herpetiformis, their families, health-care professionals and the general public.
- *Group B Strep*
  - o Group B Strep Association (GBSA)—A nonprofit organization that was formed by parents whose babies died from this devastating infection. The Group B Strep Association's goals are to educate the public

about GBS infections, promote prevention of neonatal GBS through routine prenatal screening, and promote the development of the GBS vaccine.

- *Growth Disorders*
  - o Human Growth Foundation—A voluntary, nonprofit organization whose mission is to help children and adults with disorders of growth and growth hormone through research, education, support, and advocacy.
  - o MAGIC Foundation—A national nonprofit organization created to provide support services for the families of children afflicted with a wide variety of chronic and/or critical disorders, syndromes, and diseases that affect a child's growth.
- *Guillian-Barre Syndrome*
  - o Guillian-Barre Syndrome Foundation International—Provides support and assistance to GBS patients and their families and committed to increasing knowledge and awareness in both the public and professional communities.
- *Hallervorden-Spatz Syndrome*
  - o NBIA Disorders Association—This association was created to provide families, physicians, and support providers with information about an inherited disease called Neurodegeneration with Brain Iron Accumulation (NBIA).
- *Hearing Impairment*
  - o Alexander Graham Bell Association for the Deaf and Hard of Hearing—An international membership organization and resource center on hearing loss and spoken language approaches and related issues.
  - o Wisconsin Chapter: Cochlear Implant Association, Inc.—Provides support and information and access to local support groups for adults and children who have cochlear implants, or who are interested in learning about cochlear implants.
  - o National Association for the Deaf—Programs and activities include grassroots advocacy and empowerment, captioned media, certification of American Sign Language professionals; certification of sign language interpreters; deafness-related information and publications, legal assistance, policy development and research, public awareness, and youth leadership development.
  - o National Deaf Education Network and Clearinghouse
  - o Helen Keller Services for the Blind (HKSB)—A renowned nonprofit agency with a spectrum of special services that guide legally blind New Yorkers, young and old alike, toward a life of independence and success. With its diverse services, HKSB often works one on one to

teach, educate, and rehabilitate thousands of clients according to their individual needs.

o Sign Language—Interested in sign language? Here are some great resources about American Sign Language (ASL), as well as other forms of sign language around the world.

- *Heart Disorders*
  o American Heart Association—Supports research activities broadly related to cardiovascular function and diseases, stroke, basic science, clinical, bioengineering/biotechnology and public health problems.
  o Kids with Heart National Association for Children with Heart Disorders, Inc.—Provides support, information, and education for the families of the children living with congenital heart defects and promotes public awareness of the issues that these families live with on a day-to-day basis.

- *Hemangioma*
  o National Organization of Vascular Anomalies—Dedicated to aiding individuals in the management and care of vascular anomalies.

- *Hemiplegia*
  o Alternating Hemiplegia of Childhood Foundation—Provides support to children with AHC and the parents who care for them.
  o Children's Hemiplegia and Stroke Association (CHASA)—Offers support and information to families of infants, children, and young adults who have hemiplegic cerebral palsy, hemiplegia, hemiparesis, prenatal stroke, childhood stroke, infant stroke, perinatal stroke, neonatal stroke, in utero stroke, or stroke in neonates.

- *Hemophilia*
  o National Hemophilia Foundation—Dedicated to finding better treatments and cures for bleeding and clotting disorders and to preventing the complications of these disorders through education, advocacy, and research.

- *Hemorrhagic Telangiectasia/ Osler-Weber-Rendu Syndrome*
  o Hereditary Hemorrhagic Telangiectasia (HHT) Foundation International, Inc.—A worldwide, nonprofit organization whose purpose is to support HHT patients and families and educate medical professionals.

- *Hermansky-Pudlak Syndrome*
  o Hermansky-Pudlak Syndrome (HPS) Network, Inc.—HPS is a genetic metabolic disorder which causes albinism, visual impairment, and a platelet dysfunction with prolonged bleeding. The HPS Network's mission is to gather and disseminate information, to promote awareness and research and to provide support to their members.

- *Hermaphroditism*
  - o Intersex Society of North America (ISNA)—Devoted to systemic change to end shame, secrecy, and unwanted genital surgeries for people born with an anatomy that someone decided is not standard for male or female.
- *Hernia, Diaphragmatic*
  - o CHERUBS—The Association of Congenital Diaphragmatic Hernia Research, Advocacy, and Support.
- *Histiocytosis*
  - o Histiocytosis Association of America—A nonprofit organization designed to promote scientific research, provide solutions to some of the problems specific to patients suffering from this disease, and offer support to such patients and their families and to educate and promote education related to the histiocytoses.
- *Holoprosencephaly*
  - o The Carter Centers for Brain Research—A worldwide network of scientists, health-care professionals and families dedicated to research, education, and practice.
- *Hydranencephaly*
  - o Rays of Sunshine—A comprehensive parent-driven source of information and support on the Internet available for those who care for someone with hydranencephaly. Connect with other parents who have children with hydranencephaly.
- *Hydrocephalus*
  - o Hydrocephalus Association—The Hydrocephalus Association's mission is to provide support, education, and advocacy for individuals, families, and professionals. Their goal is to ensure that families and individuals dealing with the complex issues of hydrocephalus receive personal support, comprehensive educational materials, and ongoing quality health care. They provide a wealth of services and resources to members and nonmembers alike.
  - o National Hydrocephalus Foundation—Hydrocephalus occurs when there is an imbalance between the production and the absorption of cerebral spinal fluid. The foundation website includes excellent resources and information for families.
- *Hyperlexia*
  - o American Hyperlexia Association—A nonprofit organization comprised of parents and relatives of children with hyperlexia, speech and language professionals, education professionals, and other concerned individuals with the common goal of identifying hyperlexia, promoting and facilitating effective teaching techniques both at home and

at school, and educating the general public as to the existence of the
syndrome called hyperlexia.

- *Hypoparathyroidism*
  - o National Graves' Disease Foundation—The leading cause of hyper-
    thyroidism, Graves' disease represents a basic defect in the immune
    system, causing production of immunoglobulins (antibodies) that
    stimulate and attack the thyroid gland, causing growth of the gland
    and overproduction of thyroid hormone.
- *Ichthyosis*
  - o FIRST; Foundation for Ichthyosis and Related Skin Types—Devoted to
    helping individuals and families with the genetic diseases collectively
    called the ichthyoses. Offering information and education to both lay
    and professional communities, advocating on behalf of our members in
    the political and health-care arenas and serving as a "bridge" between
    the ichthyosis community and the medical profession.
- *Immune Disorders*
  - o Immune Deficiency Foundation—Seeks to improve the diagnosis and
    treatment of patients with primary immune deficiency disease through
    research and education.
- *Incontinence*
  - o National Association for Continence (NAFC)—Leading source for
    public education and advocacy about the causes, prevention, diagno-
    sis, treatments, and management alternatives for incontinence.
- *Intestinal Pseudo-Obstruction Syndrome*
  - o International Foundation for Functional GI Disorders (IFFGD)—A
    nonprofit education and research organization whose mission is to
    inform, assist, and support people affected by GI disorders.
- *Joubert Syndrome*
  - o The Joubert Syndrome Foundation and Related Cerebellar Disor-
    ders—An international network of parents who share knowledge, ex-
    perience, and emotional support. The foundation offers a networking
    list, newsletter, and a biennial conference.
- *Kidney Disorders*
  - o American Association of Kidney Patients—Exists to serve the needs,
    interests, and welfare of all kidney patients and their families. Its mis-
    sion is to improve the lives of fellow kidney patients and their families
    by helping them deal with the physical, emotional, and social impact
    of kidney disease.
  - o National Kidney Foundation, Inc.—A major voluntary health
    organization, seeks to prevent kidney and urinary tract diseases,
    improve the health and well-being of individuals and families af-

fected by these diseases, and increase the availability of all organs for transplantation.

o Polycystic Kidney Research Foundation (PKD)—Foundation is devoted to determining the cause, improving clinical treatment, and discovering a cure.

• *Kinsborne's Syndrome*

o National Pediatric Myoclonus Center—Purpose of a national center for myoclonus is to provide the best care possible for patients whose myoclonus began during childhood.

• *Klinefelter Syndrome*

o Klinefelter Syndrome Association, Inc.—Designed to provide support and education for families and professionals dealing with the following genetic conditions: Sex chromosome variations 47XXY, 48XXYY, 48XXXY, 49XXXXY, 46XY/47XXY mosaic, and other sex chromosome variants.

• *Klippel-Trenaunay Syndrome*

o Klippel-Trenaunay Syndrome (K-T) Support Group—Welcomes patients and their families as members. This website for the K-T Support Group has been established to provide information about the group and about Klippel-Trenaunay Syndrome, and to provide families, adults with K-T, and professionals with links to the group.

• *Latex Allergy*

o Latex Allergy Information Services—Provides links to latex allergy–related websites.

• *Learning Disabilities*

o Learning Disabilities Association of America—Advocates for the almost three million students of school age with learning disabilities and for adults affected with learning disabilities.

o National Center for Learning Disabilities—Offers a periodic newsletter and educational materials for parents, educators and those with an LD.

• *Leptomeningeal Angiomatosis*

o Lesch-Nylan Registry—Offers information about genetic counseling and support groups for individuals and families with genetic conditions or birth defects, genetic counselors, clinical geneticists, and medical geneticists.

• *Leukemia*

o Leukemia and Lymphoma Society—World's largest voluntary health organization dedicated to funding blood cancer research, education, and patient services. The society's mission is to cure leukemia, lymphoma, Hodgkin's disease, and myeloma, and to improve the quality of life of patients and their families.

- *Leukodystrophy*
  - o United Leukodystrophy Foundation—Dedicated to helping children and adults who have leukodystrophy and assisting the family members, professionals, and support services that serve them. The ULF is committed to the identification, treatment, and cure of all leukodystrophies through programs of education, advocacy, research, and service.
- *Lissencephaly*
  - o Lissencephaly Network—A nonprofit organization that serves children with lissencephaly, or other neuronal migration disorder, and their families.
- *Liver Disease*
  - o American Liver Foundation—A nonprofit organization dedicated to the prevention, treatment, and cure of hepatitis and other liver diseases through research, education, and advocacy.
- *Long Q-T Syndrome*
  - o Cardiac Arrhythmias Research and Education Foundation, Inc.— Their mission is to provide funding for research and to increase professional and public awareness of unexpected sudden cardiac death due to acquired heart disease and inherited rhythm disorders.
  - o Sudden Arrhythmia Death Syndromes (SADS) Foundation— Their mission is to save the lives and support the families of children and young adults who are genetically predisposed to sudden death due to heart rhythm abnormalities.
- *Lowe Syndrome*
  - o Lowe Syndrome Association (LSA)—LSA is an international, voluntary, nonprofit organization made up of parents, friends, professionals, and others who are interested in Lowe syndrome, a rare genetic condition that affects boys.
- *Lung Diseases*
  - o American Lung Association—Fights lung disease in all its forms, with special emphasis on asthma, tobacco control, and environmental health.
- *Lupus Erthematosis*
  - o Lupus Foundation of America—Their mission is to educate and support those affected by lupus and find the cure.
  - o SLE Lupus Foundation, Inc.—Provides patient services, education, public awareness, and funding for lupus research.
- *Lyme Disease*
  - o American Lyme Disease Foundation, Inc.—A pro-active organization dedicated to the prevention, diagnosis, treatment, and control of Lyme disease and other tick-borne infections.

o Lyme Disease Foundation, Inc. (LDF)—A nonprofit medical health-care agency dedicated to finding solutions to tick-borne disorders.

- *Lymphangioma*
  o AboutFace International—Provides information and support to individuals with facial differences and their families.
- *Lymphedema*
  o National Lymphedema Network (NLN)—A nonprofit organization that provides education and guidance to lymphedema patients, health-care professionals, and the general public by disseminating information on the prevention and management of primary and secondary lymphedema.
- *Macular Diseases*
  o Association for Macular Diseases, Inc.—A not-for-profit corporation designed to promote education and research for Macular Degeneration, which is a general term used to describe a number of diseases of the retina.
  o Macular Degeneration Foundation—Dedicated to serving the interests of those affected by Macular Degeneration and related low vision conditions.
  o Macular Degeneration International—Offers information and support as its primary goal, which is done through personal contact, telephone, correspondence, Internet, and a variety of seminars and national conferences. MDI, with help from its Scientific Advisory Board also participates in research through a medical research fund, and helps to facilitate research programs by recruiting patients and families for major studies.
- *Malignant Hyperthermia*
  o Malignant Hyperthermia Association of the United States (MHAUS)—The only association in the United States dedicated to the control of malignant hyperthermia (MH). MH is a silent, inherited metabolic disorder of muscle. Affected individuals usually appear perfectly normal and have no functional difficulties in everyday life. However, when these individuals are given a triggering anesthetic this silent disorder may turn deadly.
- *Maple Syrup Urine Disease*
  o Maple Syrup Urine Disease Family Support Group—Receive general information and join the support group via their website.
- *Marfan Syndrome*
  o National Marfan Foundation—Marfan syndrome is a heritable disorder of the connective tissue that affects many organ systems, including the skeleton, lungs, eyes, heart, and blood vessels. The website is de-

signed to disseminate accurate and timely information about this condition to patients, family members, and the health-care community; to provide a network of communications for patients and relatives to share experiences, support one another, and improve their medical care; and to support and foster research.

- *Mast Cell Disease Systematic*
  o Mastocytosis Society, Inc—A nonprofit organization dedicated to helping patients, caregivers, and medical personnel understand Mast Cell Disorders and the impact they have on patient's lives.
- *Mental Illness*
  o National Alliance for the Mentally Ill (NAMI)—A nonprofit, grass-roots, self-help, support and advocacy organization of consumers, families, and friends of people with severe mental illnesses, such as schizophrenia, major depression, bipolar disorder, obsessive-compulsive disorder, and anxiety disorders.
  o SAMHSA's National Mental Health Information Center—The Substance Abuse and Mental Health Services Administration's (SAMHSA) National Mental Health Information Center provides information about mental health via a toll-free telephone number (800-789-2647), this website, and more than 600 publications. The center was developed for users of mental health services and their families, the general public, policy makers, providers, and the media.
- *Mental Retardation*
  o American Association on Intellectual and Developmental Disabilities (AAIDD)—Promotes progressive policies, sound research, effective practices, and universal human rights for people with intellectual and developmental disabilities.
  o People First International—People First and the self-advocacy movement has grown into an international movement in 43 countries, with an estimated 17,000 members or more.
  o The ARC of the United States—Advocates for the rights and full participation of all children and adults with intellectual and developmental disabilities. Together with their network of members and affiliated chapters, they improve systems of supports and services; connect families; inspire communities, and influence public policy.
- *Microcephaly*
  o FACES- The National Craniofacial Association—Dedicated to assisting children and adults who have craniofacial disorders resulting from disease, accident, or birth.
  o Genetic Alliance—An international coalition comprised of more than 600 advocacy, research, and health-care organizations that

represent millions of individuals with genetic conditions and their interests.

o March of Dimes Birth Defects Foundation—March of Dime's mission is to improve the health of babies by preventing birth defects, premature birth, and infant mortality. They carry out this mission through research, community services, education, and advocacy to save babies' lives.

* **Mitochondrial Disease**
  o United Mitochondrial Disease Foundation—Promotes research and education for the diagnosis, treatment, and cure of mitochondrial disorders and provides support to affected individuals and families.
* **MPS Disorders**
  o The National MPS Society—Mucopolysaccharidoses (MPS) and Mucolipidoses (ML) are genetic lysosomal storage disorders caused by the body's inability to produce specific enzymes. The National MPS Society supports research, supports families, and works to increase public and professional awareness.
* **Multiple Sclerosis**
  o National Multiple Sclerosis Society—The society and its network of chapters nationwide promote research, educate, advocate on critical issues, and organize a wide range of programs—including support for the newly diagnosed and those living with MS over time.
  o Multiple Sclerosis Foundation—Assistance, support, information, and resources.
* **Muscular Dystrophy**
  o Muscular Dystrophy Association—The source for news and information about neuromuscular diseases, MDA research, and services for adults and children with neuromuscular diseases and their families.
  o Muscular Dystrophy Family Foundation, Inc.—Offers comprehensive support programs to ensure clients' medical and emotional needs are taken care of. Their medical directors and case managers will help you through every stage of the process. And, the MDFF is the only agency whose mission is to fund adaptive equipment. From wheelchairs to van lifts to communication devices and beyond, they can help you get the equipment you need to live with No Boundaries® .
  o Parent Project Muscular Dystrophy—Parent Project Muscular Dystrophy mobilizes people in the United States and worldwide in a collaborative effort to enable people with Duchenne and Becker Muscular Dystrophy to survive, thrive, and fully participate within their families and communities into adulthood and beyond.

- *Myasthenia Gravis*
  - o The Myasthenia Gravis Foundation of America, Inc.—A nonprofit organization, is designed to facilitate the timely diagnosis and optimal care of individuals affected by myasthenia gravis and closely related disorders and to improve their lives through programs of patient services, public information, medical research, professional education, advocacy, and patient care.
- *Myelin Disorders*
  - o The Myelin Project—An international grassroots organization whose mission is to accelerate medical research on myelin repair.
- *Myelitis*
  - o Transverse Myelitis Association—Transverse Myelitis is a rare neurological disorder that is part of a spectrum of neuroimmunologic diseases of the central nervous system. Other disorders in this spectrum include Acute Disseminated Encephalomyelitis (ADEM), Optic Neuritis, and Neuromyelitis Optica (Devic's disease). This is an organization dedicated to advocacy for those who have these rare neuroimmunologic diseases.
- *Myeloma*
  - o International Myeloma Foundation (IMF)—The IMF is dedicated to improving the quality of life of myeloma patients while working toward prevention and a cure.
- *Myoclonus*
  - o National Pediatric Myoclonus Center—The purpose of a national center for Myoclonus is to provide the best care possible for patients whose myoclonus began during childhood.
- *Myositis Inflammatory Myopathies*
  - o The Myositis Association—Their mission is to improve the lives of those affected by inflammatory myopathies (autoimmune diseases in which the system that normally fights infections and viruses attacks healthy body tissues). They will seek out persons with inflammatory myopathies, provide a support network, act as a resource for patients and the medical community, advocate for patients, and promote research into the causes and treatment of the diseases. The Myositis Association website also includes information about Juvenile Myositis.
- *Myotubular Myopathy*
  - o Myotubular Myopathy Resource Group—This site has information about the three forms of myotubular myopathy, x-linked, autosomal recessive, and autosomal dominant. You can learn and connect with other families here and receive the periodic newsletter and other information.

- *Nager and Miller Syndromes*
  - o Foundation for Nager and Miller Syndromes (FNMS)—An international support group dedicated to helping those affected by these two similar genetic conditions that involve severe facial and limb anomalies, but does not usually affect intellect. These syndromes affect one's ability to see, hear, breathe, eat, walk, talk, and write.
- *Neurofibromatosis*
  - o Children's Tumor Foundation—A nonprofit medical foundation, dedicated to improving the health and well-being of individuals and families affected by the neurofibromatoses (NF). The neurofibromatoses (NF) are a set of genetic disorders that cause tumors to grow along various types of nerves and, in addition, can affect the development of non-nervous tissues such as bones and skin. NF causes tumors to grow anywhere on or in the body. It also leads to developmental abnormalities.
  - o Neurofibromatosis, Inc.—An organization of independent state and regional chapters, providing support and services to NF families. In addition to assisting individuals and families, NF, Inc., works closely with clinical and research professionals who specialize in the treatment of NF.
- *Neurotransmitter Disease*
  - o Pediatric Neurotransmitter Disease Association—A nonprofit, voluntary organization. The mission of the association is to help children and families who are affected by a pediatric neurotransmitter disease, support the identification of new diseases of neurotransmitter metabolism, and find better treatments and ultimately a cure for those diseases that are already known.
- *Nevi, Congenital*
  - o Nevus Network—The Congenital Nevus Support Group.
- *Niemann-Pick Disease*
  - o Ara Parseghian Medical Research Foundation—Niemann-Pick Type C disease (NP-C) is a genetic, pediatric, neurodegenerative disorder. It is responsible for the build-up of cholesterol in such areas as the spleen and liver and for accumulation of gangliosides in the brain. This ganglioside build-up results in the eventual damage to the nervous system. This metabolic disorder leads to a series of neurological problems that are ultimately fatal.
  - o National Nieman-Pick Disease Foundation, Inc.—An international, voluntary, nonprofit organization made up of parents, medical and educational professionals, friends, relatives, and others who are committed to finding a cure for Niemann-Pick disease.

- *Noonan Syndrome*
  - o Noonan Syndrome Support Group, Inc.—Noonan Syndrome is a condition that affects both children and adults. It is often associated with congenital heart disease and short stature. This group is committed to providing support, current information, and understanding to those affected by Noonan syndrome and associated anomalies.
- *Osteogenesis Imperfecta*
  - o Osteogenesis Imperfecta Foundation—The Osteogenesis Imperfecta Foundation's mission is to improve the quality of life for individuals affected by OI through research to find a cure, education, awareness, and mutual support. Osteogenesis Imperfecta (OI) is a genetic disorder characterized by bones that break easily—often from little or no apparent cause. A person with OI can break a rib while coughing, or a leg by rolling over in their sleep.
- *Ostomy*
  - o The United Ostomy Association, Inc.—The United Ostomy Association is a volunteer-based health organization dedicated to providing education, information, support, and advocacy for people who have had or will have intestinal or urinary diversions.
- *Oxalosis and Hyperoxaluria*
  - o The Oxalosis and Hyperoxaluria Foundation—The mission of the Oxalosis and Hyperoxaluria Foundation (OHF) is to seek the cause, improve the clinical treatment, and discover the cure of hyperoxaluria and oxalate stone disease and enhance the quality of life of patients and their families.
- *Pituitary Disorders*
  - o Pituitary Network Association—The Pituitary Network Association (PNA) is an international nonprofit organization for patients with pituitary tumors and disorders, their families, loved ones, and the physicians and health-care providers who treat them.
- *Polio*
  - o Post-Polio Health International—Post-Polio Health International's (PHI) mission is to enhance the lives and independence of polio survivors and home mechanical ventilator users by promoting education, networking, and advocacy among these individuals and health-care providers.
- *Prader-Willi Syndrome*
  - o Prader-Willi Association—The Prader-Willi Syndrome Association's mission is to provide to parents and professionals a national and international network of information, support services, and research endeavors to expressly meet the needs of affected children and adults and their families.

- *Pseudoxanthoma Elasticum (PXE)*
  - ○ National Association for Pseudoxanthoma Elasticum—Pseudoxanthoma Elasticum, or PXE, is an inherited disorder that affects the skin, the retina of the eyes, and the cardiovascular system.
- *Psoriasis*
  - ○ National Psoriasis Foundation—Psoriasis is a non-contagious, chronic skin disease that comes in different forms and varying levels of severity. Psoriatic arthritis is a form of joint disease that is similar to rheumatoid arthritis.
- *Reflex Sympathetic Dystrophy Syndrome*
  - ○ Reflex Sympathetic Dystrophy Syndrome Association of America—The Reflex Sympathetic Dystrophy Syndrome Association of America (RSDSA) is a national not-for-profit organization, that promotes greater public and professional awareness of RSD/CRPS, a painful neurological syndrome that may affect more than 1.5 million Americans.
- *Retinitis Pigmentosa (RP)*
  - ○ Retinitis Pigmentosa International—Under one roof, RP International offers facilities for demonstrating the latest in visual aids for the partially sighted. Information and referrals are available.
- *Rett Syndrome*
  - ○ International Rett Sydrome Association—The International Rett Syndrome Association's mission is to support and encourage research to determine the cause, treatment, and cure of; to increase public awareness of; and to provide informational and emotional support to families of children with Rett syndrome.
- *Scleroderma*
  - ○ Scleroderma Foundation—The Scleroderma Foundation is the national organization for people with scleroderma and their families and friends.
- *Scoliosis*
  - ○ Scoliosis National Foundation—The National Scoliosis Foundation (NSF) is a nonprofit organization dedicated to helping children, parents, adults, and health-care providers with the complexities of scoliosis and related spinal disorders.
- *Short Stature*
  - ○ Little People of America, Inc.—Little People of America (LPA) is a nonprofit organization that provides support and information to people of short stature and their families. On this website you'll find resources pertaining to dwarfism and LPA, medical data, instructions on how to join an e-mail discussion group, and links to numerous other dwarfism-related sites.

- *Sotos Syndrome*
  - o Sotos Syndrome Support Association—The Sotos Syndrome Support Association (SSSA) is composed of families, physicians, genetic counselors, and health-care agencies throughout the United States.
- *Speech*
  - o Apraxia Kids—Information about speech/language evaluations and how to find an experienced speech and language therapist; articles on therapy techniques written by top therapists; practical ideas and things to do at home; IQ testing and the child with apraxia; prognosis, and more.
- *Spinal Cord Injuries*
  - o Christopher and Dana Reeve Paralysis Resource Center—The Christopher and Dana Reeve Paralysis Resource Center (PRC), a program of the Christopher Reeve Paralysis Foundation (CRPF), was created in 2002 to provide a comprehensive, national source of information for people living with paralysis and their caregivers to promote health, foster involvement in the community, and improve quality of life. This site has a "kids-only area."
- *Spinal Muscular Atrophy*
  - o Families of Spinal Muscular Atrophy—Families of Spinal Muscular Atrophy is the largest international organization dedicated solely to eradicating spinal muscular atrophy (SMA) by promoting and supporting research, helping families cope with SMA through informational programs and support, and educating the public and professional community about SMA.
- *Spina Bifida*
  - o Spina Bifida Assoc. of America—The mission of the Spina Bifida Association of America is to promote the prevention of spina bifida and to enhance the lives of all affected.
- *Stickler Syndrome*
  - o Stickler Involved People—Stickler syndrome is a connective tissue disorder, a genetic malfunction in the tissue that connects bones, heart, eyes, and ears. This disorder is associated with problems of vision, hearing, bone and joint, facial and cleft palate, and heart.
- *Stroke*
  - o National Stroke Association—The National Stroke Association (NSA) provides education, services, and community-based activities in prevention, treatment, rehabilitation, and recovery. NSA serves the public and professional communities, people at risk, patients and their health-care providers, stroke survivors, and their families and caregivers.

- *Sturge-Weber Syndrome*
  o The Sturge-Weber Foundation—The Sturge-Weber Foundation's mission is to improve the quality of life for individuals with Port Wine Stains (PWS), Sturge-Weber Syndrome (SWS), and Klippel-Trenaunay Syndrome (KT). The foundation strives to meet this goal by providing worldwide education and support and by facilitating research that could ultimately lead to a cure.
- *Stuttering*
  o Stuttering Foundation of America—The Stuttering Foundation provides free online resources, services, and support to those who stutter and their families, as well as support for research into the causes of stuttering.
  o The National Center for Stuttering—The purpose of the National Center for Stuttering is to provide up-to-date factual information about stuttering, to provide a National Stutterer's Hotline, to treat small groups of selected individuals who stutter, to provide continuing education for speech pathologists, and to conduct research into the causes and treatment of stuttering.
- *Sudden Arrhythmia Death Syndromes*
  o Sudden Arrhythmia Death Syndromes Foundation—The SADS Foundation is committed to supporting families and individuals with genetically mediated cardiac arrhythmias through education, research, and advocacy.
- *Sudden Infant Death Syndrome*
  o Back to Sleep Campaign—Information on the Healthy Child Care Back to Sleep Campaign.
  o National SIDS Resource Center—The National Sudden Infant Death Syndrome Resource Center (NSRC) provides information services and technical assistance on sudden infant death syndrome (SIDS) and related topics.
- *Tay-Sachs Disease*
  o The National Tay-Sachs and Allied Diseases Association (NTSAD)—The National Tay-Sachs and Allied Diseases Association (NTSAD) is dedicated to the treatment and prevention of Tay-Sachs, Canavan, and related diseases, and to provide information and support services to individuals and families affected by these diseases, as well as the public at large. Strategies for achieving these goals include public and professional education, research, genetic screening, family services, and advocacy.
- *Tourette Syndrome*
  o Tourette Syndrome Association—The Tourette Syndrome Association's mission is to identify the cause of, find the cure for, and control the effects of this disorder.

- **Tremor**
  - o International Essential Tremor Foundation—The International Essential Tremor Foundation (IETF) was created to provide information, services, and support to individuals and families affected by essential tremor (ET). The organization encourages and promotes research in an effort to determine the causes, treatment, and ultimately the cure for ET.
- **Trisomy 18, 13**
  - o Support Organization for Trisomy 18, 13, and Related Disorders (SOFT)—SOFT is a nonprofit volunteer organization offering support for parents who have had a child with a chromosome disorder, and education to families and professionals interested in the care of these children.
  - o Turner Syndrome Society of the United States—The Turner Syndrome Society of the United States works to provide a public forum for communication of state-of-the-art information, exchange of ideas, and social support and strives to increase public awareness of Turner syndrome, its effects, and its possibilities.
- **Tuberous Sclerosis**
  - o Tuberous Sclerosis Alliance—The Tuberous Sclerosis Alliance is dedicated to finding a cure for Tuberous Sclerosis while improving the lives of those affected.
- **Urea Cycle Disorders**
  - o National Urea Cycle Disorders Foundation—The National Urea Cycle Disorders Foundation is a nonprofit organization dedicated to the identification, treatment, and cure of urea cycle disorders. A urea cycle disorder is a genetic disorder caused by a deficiency of one of the enzymes in the urea cycle, which is responsible for removing ammonia from the blood stream.
- **Vestibular Disorders**
  - o The Vestibular Disorders Association—VEDA is a nonprofit organization that provides information to the public about inner-ear balance disorders such as Meniere's disease, BPPV, and labyrinthitis. Symptoms of vestibular disorders may include dizziness, imbalance, vertigo, nausea, and fuzzy vision and may be accompanied by hearing problems.
- **Visual Impairments**
  - o American Council of the Blind—The American Council of the Blind strives to improve the well-being of all blind and visually impaired people by serving as a representative national organization of blind people; elevating the social, economic, and cultural levels of blind

people; improving educational and rehabilitation facilities and opportunities; cooperating with the public and private institutions and organizations concerned with blind services; encouraging and assisting all blind persons to develop their abilities; and conducting a public education program to promote greater understanding of blindness and the capabilities of blind people.

o American Foundation for the Blind—The American Foundation for the Blind is dedicated to addressing the critical issues of literacy, independent living, employment, and access through technology for the ten million Americans who are blind or visually impaired.

o Aurora Ministries—Offers free audio Bibles for the blind and print handicapped in approximately 70 languages.

o Braille Institute of America—The Braille Institute is a nonprofit organization dedicated to eliminating blindness and severe sight loss.

o Lighthouse International—Lighthouse International is dedicated to fighting vision loss through prevention, treatment, and empowerment.

o National Federation for the Blind—Contains information on Braille, guide dogs, convention reports, legislation for the blind, literature for the blind, and other services.

o Recording for the Blind and Dyslexic—For more than 50 years, RFB&D has been an invaluable educational resource, enabling those with print disabilities to complete their educations, advance their careers, and gain self-esteem.

• *Vitiligo*
  o National Vitiligo Foundation—This site was created to serve as a clearinghouse for information about vitiligo, for both people with vitiligo and the general public. Vitiligo is spontaneous irregular depigmentation of skin, which can occur at any stage in life.

• *Von Hippel-Lindau Syndrome*
  o VHL Family Alliance Homepage—Dedicated to improving diagnosis, treatment, and quality of life for individuals and families affected by von Hippel-Lindau disease.

• *Williams Syndrome*
  o Williams Syndrome Association—The Williams Syndrome Foundation (WSF) seeks to create or enhance opportunities in education, housing, employment, and recreation for people who have Williams Syndrome and other related or similar conditions. The WSF identifies, initiates, funds and provides strategic guidance for major, long-range development projects, either by itself, or by cooperating with other organizations.

WOUNDED WARRIORS

When battlefield injury occurs far from home, the road to recovery may be long and difficult to navigate. Even with the dedicated support of medical professionals, loved ones, military leadership, and brothers- and sisters-in-arms, this pathway from injury to home requires caring over time and over miles. Differences in the type of injury, in the nature of support available along the way, and the types of resources and responsibilities waiting at home may dictate different stops along the way for different service members.

Movement from care at the point of battlefield injury—physical, psychological, or combined—through levels of care abroad and within the United States and ultimately homeward is a complex process involving the interplay of personal endurance, military and medical leadership, technology and communications, and networks of civilian and military caregivers, supporters, and communities. The modern evacuation and movement of the injured provides new opportunities for care, necessary tracking and communications, and needs for protection from additional health burdens, both physical and administrative.

1. More than 75,000 service members have sustained combat injury in the wars in Iraq and Afghanistan. Approximately half of these have been serious enough that the service member has been unable to continue to function in theater and has required a medical evacuation back to the continental United States. The injuries include but are by no means limited to traumatic amputations, loss of sight, and traumatic brain injury. The emotionally injured may also be evacuated. Important, even severe emotional injuries may not be readily apparent on the battlefield and occur in greater numbers as home approaches and the challenges of return meet the worries of lost health and function.
2. The "invisibility" of psychological injury presents a complex medical situation in which denial, stigma, fear of re-exposure to painful memories, and lack of knowledge of treatment options and efficacy impede help-seeking and strain an already stressed system of care resources. Administrative procedures can become part of secondary injury. At the same time, when health systems create opportunities to miss care, the combination of fears, stigma, and emotional pain can enhance missed opportunities for psychological and behavioral care.
3. Most serious combat injuries powerfully impact the children and families of service members. Longitudinal data suggest that problems do not immediately resolve and commonly worsen during the course of the first year after hospitalization. Difficulty in readjusting to life

back home may alter family relationships and support, contributing to a vicious cycle of psychosocial challenges for both the injured service member and the family. The family should be seen as care collaborators in all health interventions and planning.

4. Returning combat veterans, even those not psychologically injured, experience a variety of behavioral and emotional responses secondary to their war experience. Distress symptoms are common and may include insomnia, nightmares, or other forms of sleep disorder; hypervigilance, jitteriness or overexcitement; and avoidance or social withdrawal. Reintegration with family and life is a goal and can be a challenge.

5. Systems of care must address not only disorders, but also the many emotional and behavioral manifestations of distress. They must incorporate health care provided by military, VA, and civilian treatment facilities; facilitate family participation in health care and treatment planning; and engage traditional community resources (e.g., churches and schools) as well as employee and local, state, and federal programs implemented specifically to provide assistance to returning veterans.

6. Secondary injury can result from the induced helplessness, overwhelming stress, and indignities resulting from administrative delays, errors, and omissions, which may unnecessarily complicate recovery.

7. Variability in the time and emotional availability and responsiveness of family members requires resources and flexibility in order to identify and establish care advocates for each injured service member.

8. People returning from combat deployment can sometimes initiate or increase the frequency of risk behaviors that compromise their health and the health and safety of those around them. Excessive alcohol use may develop as a misguided attempt to reduce stress. Irritability or anger (common symptoms on return home) may turn into violence, at times directed to one's family, in the context of excessive alcohol use or the decreased emotional control that can accompany Traumatic Brain Injury.

9. Medical advances and current practice have altered the amount of time an individual may remain in a specific care environment. Rarely in the modern world of war is the injured now in theater or even overseas for long periods of time. Yet healing and administrative processes still take time and hold patients in new settings where family may or may not be present and resources have to be constantly adjusted to meet needs. Resources have to be sufficient and flexibly assigned to meet each level of care in order to sustain the recovery process and be responsive to the cultural context of the injured and geographical considerations (i.e., those residing in rural or remote locations).

10. Current processes of medical evacuation generally provide for superb initial stabilization and management of physical and psychosocial injuries to service members within the military medical system. However they do not well address the longer-term challenges associated with care across boundaries of community, family, and VA and civilian medical services. The care of injured from battlefield to home must be re-engineered to incorporate the new health care available, the technology and transport and the varied effects of injury on family members, the subsequent impact on the nature and availability of family resources to the injured service member, and the range in available resources during evacuation and at home station over time.

11. Navigating the complexities of ongoing medical care and disability evaluation is in and of itself a health challenge and a health burden. It can be an impediment to the intrinsically human process of adaptation to serious physical or emotional injury. Navigating this complex road requires acknowledging the injury's impact on one's identity, one's future, one's family, and one's livelihood. Such knowledge changes how we view ourselves and our family, and can change how our family and friends view us and our future. This adaptation, recovery, and return requires time and community to sustain the process.

Injured service members are often treated at medical facilities a great distance away from their homes. The military recognizes the benefits of a family's visit while a service member recuperates and often provides assistance in transporting family members to the facility where the service member is recuperating. In addition, a number of private organizations provide further travel assistance to qualified family members. These organizations include the Fisher House Foundation, which provides free or low-cost lodgings at Fisher Houses located on the grounds of military and VA medical centers throughout the country, as well as free airline tickets through its Hero Miles program. In addition, family members who need time off from work to be with a recuperating service member may benefit from the Family and Medical Leave Act (FMLA), a federal law that guarantees many workers up to 12 weeks of unpaid leave during a 12-month period to care for family members suffering from serious medical conditions.

The financial consequences of an injury are generally not the first concern for service members and their families. However, understanding the various benefits available to assist with financial needs is an important part of the recovery process. Service members, including reservists, may continue to receive full pay while recovering from injury and awaiting a medical evaluation. In addition, a program called Traumatic Servicemembers' Group Life Insurance (TSGLI) provides qualified service members with assistance in the direct aftermath of a severe injury. Coverage is retroactive to qualifying service members who suffered traumatic injuries in Iraq and Afghanistan on or after October 7, 2001.

Casualty Status

According to the DoD, a casualty is "any person who is lost to the organization by reason of having been declared beleaguered, besieged, captured, dead, diseased, detained, duty status whereabouts unknown, injured, ill, interned, missing, missing in action, or wounded."

When a service member is injured, gets sick, or is hospitalized, he or she becomes a "casualty." The service member is then further categorized according to his/her casualty type and the casualty status.

The military now categorizes casualties as dead, wounded, ill, or injured with subdivisions such as very seriously ill or injured, seriously ill or injured, and not seriously ill or injured. Originally the DoD categories only covered combat casualties but these have now been expanded to cover all injuries and illnesses. The new categories now take into account many other conditions, including psychological and traumatic injuries as a result of wars.

Federal Recovery Coordinators

Federal recovery coordinators ensure the appropriate oversight and coordination are provided for care of active duty service members and veterans with major amputations, severe traumatic brain injury, spinal cord injury, severe sight or hearing impairments, and severe multiple injuries. The coordinators also work closely with family members to take care of services and needs. The aim is to ensure that lifelong medical and rehabilitative care services and other federal benefits are provided to seriously wounded, injured, and ill active duty service members, veterans, and their families.

The coordinators have a background in health-care management and work closely with the clinicians and case management teams to develop and execute plans of services needed across the continuum of care, from recovery through rehabilitation to reintegration to civilian life.

These federal recovery coordinators ensure a smooth transition of wounded service members through the VA's health-care system, while also cutting red tape for other benefits.

Your Support Team

Wounded service members have case managers assigned to work with them during their recovery period. The job of these individuals is to provide information and help assist the service member and family during the recovery period and the Physical Evaluation Board (PEB) and Medical Evaluation Board (MEB) process. These individuals also provide information on Veteran Service Organizations (VSOs). Many military hospitals serving wounded or injured service members also have Family Assistance Centers. Liaison officers also serve in hospitals acting as the advocate for the patient and the link between the wounded warriors and their units and families. The liaison officer also works with patient administrative teams who help gather patient treatment information, make travel arrangements, connect with the families, and act as a link with charitable organizations.

Families can also seek assistance from installation chaplains, social workers, and family centers: Army Community Services, Marine Corps Community Services, Air Force Family Support Center, Navy Fleet and Family Support Center, and Coast Guard Work Life Offices.

Military bodies responsible for assisting injured service members and wounded transitioning veterans:

Army—Wounded Warrior Transition Brigades
Navy—Safe Harbor Program
Marine Corps—Marine for Life and Wounded Warrior Regiment
Air Force—Palace HART (Helping Airmen Recover Together)

Important note: The wars in Iraq and Afghanistan have resulted in tens of thousands of wounded warriors and this has put additional pressures and strains on military marriages. In many cases this has also brought about a significant change in the spousal role. Partners who used to stay at home are now caregivers as well but may have to consider becoming the bread winner. While the wounded warrior is entitled to a whole range of benefits and help, it may still not be enough to pay all the bills. In such cases, spouses may have to consider getting a job or going back to school to get new qualifications. If you have been out of the workforce for some time, it can be very challenging searching out new jobs, doing the rounds of interviews, getting your resume up-to-date, and so on. Fortunately help is available for all of these things with guidance on job hunting, available work and even resume writing.

Please also see *The Wounded Warrior Handbook* by Don Philpott, Janelle Hill, and Cheryl Lawhorne, published by Government Institutes. It is an easy-to-use, comprehensive reference guide for wounded warriors, as well as for their families and loved ones. There is a huge and growing amount of literature available from the military and others; there are scores of support organizations involved in this arena and there are hundreds of websites offering information and help. All of these do a magnificent job in their respective areas, but it can be a daunting task to pull together all this information, especially at a time of crisis. The information in this handbook was gathered from hundreds of these sources and resources in the public domain and elsewhere and includes the most up-to-date information about health services and benefits from the Department of Veterans Affairs. The handbook also deals with other critical issues such as important financial, legal, and tax matters, although this is provided purely as guidance. The handbook provides a comprehensive framework that will allow wounded warriors and their families to quickly access information they need regarding medical treatment, rehabilitation, counseling, support, and transition.

A Family Member's Trauma

From the moment you were informed that your service member was deploying into a combat zone, your life altered. The normal routine shifted to include the underlying concern felt when a loved one is in harm's way. The day you received notification that your service member was wounded, you were wounded as well. Families are connected: what happens to one member affects all the other members of the family. While attention is focused on supporting your service member, time needs to be spent as well acknowledging your own traumatic experience, and the ongoing effects this experience will have on you and your life.

Notification can be a traumatic experience in and of itself. Even when you know that your service member is in a combat zone and anything can happen, it is still a shock when you receive a phone call stating that something has. That phone call triggers a series of events that eventually lead you to travel from the comfort of your home to the unfamiliar hospital bedside of your service member. Travel, even under the best of circumstances, is a stressful event. When combined with reuniting with your seriously wounded service member it becomes even more so. All these experiences in such a short amount of time can be overwhelming, and then you begin to factor in the reality of the injuries and condition of your service member. Life can suddenly feel out of control.

Whether you are a spouse, parent, child, or other relative of the service member, your life has been irrevocably changed by the events that brought you here. Change is a challenging thing and often uncomfortable while you adapt to the new reality the change has brought to your life. With change, something of the old way of life is lost, and as with all loss, there is a normal period when grieving occurs. No one can know what your loss is. Each of us is unique, and what may be significant to one person may not be to another.

Your grieving process is personal. Take some time to think about what you have lost.

Acknowledge your own loss and grieve for it. Understand that the extent of your own loss is not fully apparent now. It will take time to realize how much your life will be changed by this experience. Be patient with yourself while you come to grips with the shift in your life.

Your trauma is real. While you might tell yourself it is nothing compared to what your service member is enduring, it will have an effect on you. Being aware of that gives you some measure of control to lessen that effect. You have the right to feel pain and sorrow. Take care of yourself. Focus on what you have the power to do: that is, to change your own actions or reactions. Actively pursue stress management. Utilize the resources available to you. Seek out and utilize support services for yourself and your children. The social worker assigned to your service member is there for you as well. Your entire family has been wounded along with your service member, and it deserves the same care and concern as you are giving your service member.

WAR ZONE–RELATED STRESS REACTIONS: WHAT FAMILIES NEED TO KNOW

A National Center for PTSD Fact Sheet

Military personnel in war zones frequently have serious reactions to their traumatic war experiences. Sometimes the reactions continue after they return home. Ongoing reactions to war-zone fear, horror, or helplessness are connected to posttraumatic stress and can include:

- Nightmares or difficulty sleeping
- Unwanted distressing memories or thoughts
- Anxiety and panic
- Irritability and anger
- Emotional numbing or loss of interest in activities or people
- Problem alcohol or drug use to cope with stress reactions

How Traumatic Stress Reactions Can Affect Families

- Stress reactions may interfere with a service member's ability to trust and be emotionally close to others. As a result, families may feel emotionally cut off from the service member.
- A returning war veteran may feel irritable and have difficulty communicating, which may make it hard to get along with him or her.

- A returning veteran may experience a loss of interest in family social activities.
- Veterans with PTSD may lose interest in sex and feel distant from their spouses.
- Traumatized war veterans often feel that something terrible may happen "out of the blue" and can become preoccupied with trying to keep themselves and family members safe.
- Just as war veterans are often afraid to address what happened to them, family members are frequently fearful of examining the traumatic events as well. Family members may want to avoid talking about the trauma or related problems. They may avoid talking because they want to spare the survivor further pain or because they are afraid of his or her reaction.
- Family members may feel hurt, alienated, or discouraged because the veteran has not been able to overcome the effects of the trauma. Family members may become angry or feel distant from the veteran.

The Important Role of Families in Recovery

The primary source of support for the returning service member is likely to be his or her family.

Families can help the veteran not withdraw from others. Families can provide companionship and a sense of belonging, which can help counter the veteran's feeling of separateness because of his or her experiences. Families can provide practical and emotional support for coping with life stressors.

If the veteran agrees, it is important for family members to participate in treatment. It is also important to talk about how the posttraumatic stress is affecting the family and what the family can do about it. Adult family members should also let their loved ones know that they are willing to listen if the service member would like to talk about war experiences. Family members should talk with treatment providers about how they can help in the recovery effort.

What Happens in Treatment for PTSD?

Treatment for PTSD focuses on helping the trauma survivor reduce fear and anxiety, gain control over traumatic stress reactions, make sense of war experiences, and function better at work and in the family. A standard course of treatment usually includes:

- Assessment and development of an individual treatment plan.

- Education of veterans and their families about posttraumatic stress and its effects.
- Training in relaxation methods, to help reduce physical arousal/tension.
- Practical instruction in skills for coping with anger, stress, and ongoing problems.
- Detailed discussion of feelings of anger or guilt, which are very common among survivors of war trauma.
- Detailed discussions to help change distressing beliefs about self and others (e.g., self-blame).
- If appropriate, careful, repeated discussions of the trauma (exposure therapy) to help the service member reduce the fear associated with trauma memories.
- Medication to reduce anxiety, depression, or insomnia.
- Group support from other veterans is often felt to be the most valuable treatment experience.

Mental health professionals in VA medical centers, community clinics, and Readjustment Counseling Service Vet Centers have a long tradition of working with family members of veterans with PTSD. Couples counseling and educational classes for families may be available. Family members can encourage the survivor to seek education and counseling, but should not try to force their loved one to get help. Family members should consider getting help for themselves, whether or not their loved one is getting treatment.

Self-Care Suggestions for Families

- Become educated about PTSD.
- Take time to listen to all family members and show them that you care.
- Spend time with other people. Coping is easier with support from others, including extended family, friends, church groups, or other community groups.
- Join or develop a support group.
- Take care of yourself. Family members frequently devote themselves totally to those they care for and, in the process, neglect their own needs. Pay attention to yourself. Watch your diet and exercise, and get plenty of rest. Take time to do things that feel good to you.
- Try to maintain family routines, such as dinner together, church, or sports outings.
- If needed, get professional help as early as possible, and get back in touch with treatment providers if things worsen after treatment has ended.

For more information about PTSD please visit the VA website at www. va.gov.

A PTSD guide for families can be found at
www.helpguide.org/mental/post_traumatic_stress_disorder_symptoms_ treatment.html.

3

Caregiving and Support

DEMANDS OF BEING A PRIMARY CAREGIVER

Stress

Many service members who have experienced combat, and their families, are familiar with the term "combat stress." The effects of combat, however, aren't limited to those directly connected to the experience. Stress can affect anyone who cares for those individuals.

America Supports You is a Defense Department program connecting citizens and corporations with military personnel and their families serving at home and abroad.

"One of the things that we've learned from experience and research is that 'compassion fatigue,' and the potential for burning out, is not just limited to psychotherapists," said Dr. Joseph Bobrow, executive director of the Coming Home Project. "Family members who are caring for wounded veterans are at risk. Veteran service workers, like yourselves, [and] volunteers [are at risk]." Becoming overwhelmed by the experience of caring for service members and their families is the nature of that work. "We can anticipate this happening," he said. "It doesn't necessarily . . . mean a psychiatric disorder, just like post-traumatic stress . . . is not necessarily a psychiatric disorder. In fact, it's the body, mind and soul's way of coping with an impossible situation," he explained. Burnout, or compassion fatigue, can be overcome, but it's better to avoid it to begin with, he said. Incorporating positive thoughts and actions into daily life builds resiliency against burnout.

COUNSELING AND SUPPORT SYSTEMS

Life in the military is challenging. When you have a child with special needs it is even more so. However, families in the military have a vast array of resources available to them, from within and beyond the military community. Help yourself and your family by learning about the support services and resources that are available.

Military Community Resources

Family Support Centers (FSC) are there to help military families. Most military installations have one or more FSCs that offer a variety of free services and support designed to assist service members and their families with the unique challenges of military life. Available offerings may vary due to the size and mission of the installation. Types of assistance may include the following:

Relocation counseling and lending lockers
Information and referrals for special needs
Employment workshops
Volunteer coordination
Parenting classes
Individual and family counseling
Personal finance management
Spouse education and support programs
Deployment support
Family life education and workshops

Family Support Centers can connect you with the Exceptional Family Member Program. This will ensure that your child's medical and educational needs will be considered as a duty station is selected.

Your FSC is also a good place to ask for information about local organizations and support groups concerned with specific disabilities. To find the Family Support Center nearest you, go to www.militaryinstallations.dod.mil.

New Parent Support Program

The New Parent Support Program (www.militaryhomefront.dod.mil) assists expectant and new parents through a variety of services. Services are matched to the needs of individual families and include home visitations, education, counseling, and referrals to other resources to include special needs organizations and services aboard the installation and within the local community. Parents who take advantage of the classes offered will gain hands on training that will help them make informed and responsible decisions for their children.

Family Advocacy Program (FAP)

The military community is not immune to personal or family problems. Problems may range from experiencing stress due to a deployment to experiencing domestic violence including spouse or child abuse. Fortunately, vital services and support are available to military families. FAP sponsors activities and services to include public awareness briefings, individual and couples counseling, crisis intervention, support groups, stress management, and other well-being workshops. FAP services may be found at military medical facilities or at installation Family Support Centers.

Child, Youth, and Teen Development Programs

Military families face greater challenges than most other families. Shifting work schedules that are often longer than the typical 8-hour day and the obligation to be ready to deploy anywhere in the world on a moment's notice requires a child development system that is flexible, yet maintains high standards. Add to these challenges a child with special needs, and finding quality child care can be a formidable challenge.

Child Development Centers. DoD Child Development Centers (CDCs) provide care for children 6 weeks to 12 years of age. To help ensure the needs of your exceptional child are met in the daycare setting, the Army, Navy, and Marine Corps offer special needs resource teams. Contact information for all DoD CDCs is available at www.defense.gov.

Family Child Care (FCC). FCC homes operated on base are certified by the military child development program. These providers deliver critical services to service members on shift work, working extended hours or weekends, and for those who prefer a home-based environment for their children. A family child care home may be the best option for special needs children who need the consistency of a single caregiver or who require complex procedures that must be learned by the caregiver.

Youth Centers. Ask about available youth programs at your FSC. You will find an array of programs that will help your child become involved and make friends. Frequently available are sports leagues for soccer, basketball, and baseball and a center where your child can play Ping-Pong or video games. For information regarding Child Youth and Teen Services see www.militaryhomefront.dod.mil.

Summer Camps and Recreation.   Several bases have special camps and activities for children with special needs. Camp Lejeune offers *Camp Special Time* several weekends a year, giving parents some well-deserved time off. Fort Campbell offers *Camp We Can.* Ask about what is available on your base and in your community.

School Liaison Officers

The Army sponsors a program providing a school liaison officer at each Army installation whose role is to work with local schools in support of children from military families. The School Liaison Officer is particularly helpful when a student is transitioning from one school system to another and may be able to advocate on the parents' behalf when they believe their child's special education needs are not being met. For more information about this program, go to www.militarystudent.dod.mil.

Relief Societies

Military communities pride themselves on taking care of their own. Relief societies exist to help families with unexpected problems or financial emergencies. Help may be available for the following needs:

Emergency transportation
Funeral expenses
Disaster relief assistance
Child care expenses
Essential vehicle repairs
Unforeseen family emergencies
Food, rent, and utilities
Medical/dental bills (patient's share)

Each of the Armed Forces has established its own relief society.

Army Emergency Relief Society
www.aerhq.org
1-866-878-6378
Navy/Marine Corps Relief Society
1-703-696-4904
Air Force Aid Society
www.afas.org
1-800-769-8951

Service-Sponsored Websites

Each branch of the military sponsors a website that provides an overview of programs and support available to military personnel and family members. These websites also provide news articles and information relating to life in the military and online tutorials.

U.S. Army
MyArmyLifeToo.com
www.myarmylifetoo.com
U.S. Navy
LIFELines Services Network
www.lifelines.navy.mil
U.S. Marine Corps
Marine Corps Community Services
www.usmc-mccs.org
U.S. Air Force
Air Force Cross Roads
www.afcrossroads.com

Additional Military Resources

MilitaryHOMEFRONT's Special Needs/EFMP Module

MilitaryHOMEFRONT's (www.militaryhomefront.dod.mil/efm) Special Needs/EFMP module is the Official Department of Defense website that was designed to help troops and their family members who have special needs. This site is packed with information. MilitaryHOMEFRONT maintains a Military Community Directory that has a searchable list of family center addresses, websites, phone numbers, and e-mail addresses worldwide. Here you will also find resources to support the following:

Exceptional Family Member Program
Parenting
Relocation
Tip sheets
Military Spouse Resource Center
Military Saver
List of benefits and services
Pre-separation guide
Military Teens on the Move
General legal information

Deployment connections
Employment and transition assistance

Military OneSource

Military OneSource (www.militaryonesource.com) provides information, referrals, and assistance to the military community. Accessed by telephone or the Internet, Military OneSource provides special needs consultation, research, resources, and materials intended to enhance current military services available to families with special needs.

A Military Education Specialist is available and devoted to military families who need assistance with issues related to educating their children. Services are provided on a scheduled appointment basis via telephone and are focused on special needs children ages birth to 21. Specialty services can be accessed through the main telephone number for Military One-Source, and an appointment with a military special needs specialist should be requested.

Many tip sheets covering a wide range of topics of interest to military families with needs are available. All services are free of charge.

Military Teens on the Move (MTOM)

MTOM (www.dod.mil/mtom) is a website specifically for military teens and kids who are facing yet another move. Here they will find age appropriate information about how to deal with the feelings they have about moving, information about the new installation, and advice on handling the move and how to begin to fit in at their new home.

PlanMyMove

This is a comprehensive moving tool that includes tools for military families with special needs. It lets you create customized moving tools such as calendars, to do lists, and arrival checklists, all intended to help you get organized and to make your next move as smooth as possible.

TRICARE

TRICARE offers several programs to assist families with special needs. Extended Care Health Option (ECHO) offers financial assistance and additional benefits for services, equipment, or supplies beyond those available through TRICARE Prime, Extra, or Standard. Also available is ECHO Home Health

Care (EHHC). EHHC provides homebound family members with intensive home health care services.

Federal, State, and Community Resources

American Red Cross

Today's American Red Cross is keeping pace with the changing military. The Red Cross sends communications on behalf of family members who are facing emergencies or other important events to members of the U.S. Armed Forces serving all over the world. Both active duty and community-based military can count on the Red Cross to provide access to financial assistance, counseling and assistance to veterans, and emergency communications that link them with their families back home. Contact the Red Cross at www. redcross.org or 1-202-303-4498.

Computer/Electronics Accommodations Program (CAP)

The Computer/Electronic Accommodations Program provides assistive technology and services to people with disabilities, federal managers, supervisors, IT professionals, and wounded service members. "We buy it, we pay for it, we get it to the users, it's just that simple," says Dinah Cohen, CAP Director. You can find additional information about CAP's EFMP initiatives at or call 1-703-681-8813 (voice) or 1-703-681-0881 (tty).

Disabilityinfo.gov

This website, www.disabilityinfo.gov, connects people with disabilities to the information and resources they need to pursue their personal and professional ambitions. Disabled individuals can look here for information about travel, workplace support, and fair housing.

Cadre (National Center on Dispute Resolution)

Cadre encourages the use of mediation and other collaborative strategies to resolve disagreements about special education and early intervention programs. Cadre offers a spectrum of services including promoting ways to prevent conflict and help with early dispute assistance, education about conflict resolution options, mediation, resolution sessions, and due process hearings. To contact Cadre, go to www.directionservice.org or call 1-541-686-5060 (voice) or 1-541-284-4740 (tty) or send a fax to 1-541-686-5063.

Food Stamps and FSSA

The Food Stamp Program (www.fns.usda.gov) serves as the first line of defense against hunger. It enables low-income families to buy nutritious food with Electronic Benefits Transfer (EBT) cards. Food stamp recipients spend their benefits to buy eligible food in authorized retail food stores, including the commissary. To pre-qualify online, go to the website and click on "Pre Screening Tool."

Food stamps are not available for military families stationed overseas. However, you can apply for the Family Subsistence Supplemental Allowance (FSSA). Although this allowance does target those families currently using food stamps, all total force members may apply because it is based on household income and family size, not whether one is currently receiving food stamps. Nothing in the law prohibits service members from receiving both FSSA and food stamp benefits at the same time. However, the FSP will count any FSSA benefits as income, just like any other military income, in determining eligibility and allotment amounts under the FSP. For more information, go to www.dmdc.osd.mil.

Medicaid

Medicaid (www.cms.hhs.gov) is a program that pays for health care for some individuals and families with low income and few resources. Medicaid is a national program with broad guidelines, but each state sets its own eligibility rules and decides what services to provide. Be aware of this as you move from state to state. In most states, children who qualify for Social Security Income (SSI) will also qualify for Medicaid. States can also choose to cover other groups of children under the age of 19 or those who live in higher income families.

Many states qualify children though programs that allow disabled children to qualify without considering their parents' income. To find information on Medicaid and Medicaid waivers in your state go to www.cms.hhs.gov.

National Center on Education, Disability, and Juvenile Justice (EDJJ)

EDJJ is concerned about the number of youth with disabilities at risk for contact with the courts or already involved in the juvenile delinquency system. They provide assistance, conduct research, and disseminate resources in three areas: prevention of school failure and delinquency, education and special education for detained and committed youth, and transition services for youth returning to schools and communities. For more information go to www.edjj.org or call 1-301-405-6462.

NICHCY

NICHCY (www.nichcy.org) has a wealth of information on disabilities. NICHCY stands for the National Dissemination Center for Children with Disabilities and serves the nation as a central source of information on the following:

Disabilities in infants, toddlers, children, and youth
IDEA, which is the law authorizing special education
No Child Left Behind (as it relates to children with disabilities)
Research-based effective educational practices

NICHCY is a valuable resource for all parents of disabled children and is linked to the BrowseAloud text reader. This means all the information on this site can be read to you.

Shriners Hospitals for Children

Shriners Hospitals are a network of 22 pediatric hospitals in the United States, Canada, and Mexico that provide specialized care for orthopedic conditions, burns, spinal cord injuries, and cleft lip and palate. All services are provided at no charge.

If you know of a child Shriners Hospitals might be able to help, please call the toll-free patient referral line.

In the U.S.: 1-800-237-5055
In Canada: 1-800-361-7256.

Specialized Training of Military Parents

STOMP is the only National Parent Training and Information Center for military families that provides support and advice to military parents regardless of the type of medical condition their child has. The STOMP Project hosts a list serve for military families and professionals to use to share ideas. The list serve enables military families all over the world to connect, learn, and help each other as they raise their special needs children in military communities.

On STOMP parents can ask questions and get answers about the resources available to them, as well as receive advice on educating their children and navigating the health-care system. STOMP offers workshops addressing an array of topics. You can contact STOMP at www.stompproject.org or 1-800-5-PARENT (v/tty).

Supplemental Security Income (SSI)

SSI (www.ssa.gov) is a federal supplement program that can provide a monthly payment to those with low incomes and few resources who are 65 or older, blind, or disabled. Children may qualify. If you think you or your child might qualify, visit the nearest Social Security Office or call the Social Security Administration Office at 1-800-772-1213. If the application is denied, it is a good practice to appeal the decision.

Women, Infants, and Children (WIC)

The WIC website (www.fns.usda.gov) has a link to toll-free numbers across the country. If you can't access the Internet, call the state Nutrition Counseling office or nearest military family support center. WIC offers nutritional help to women and children who are low-income and nutritionally at risk. This includes women who are pregnant, postpartum, or breast-feeding, and infants and children up to their fifth birthday. WIC provides nutrition education, nutritious foods, as well as screening and referrals to other health, welfare, and social services.

Service members living overseas may be eligible to participate in the WIC Overseas program. For more information about this program, go to www.tricare.mil.

Wrightslaw

Parents, educators, advocates, and attorneys go to Wrightslaw (www.wrightslaw.com) for reliable information about special education law and advocacy for children with disabilities. Wrightslaw includes thousands of articles, cases, and free resources on dozens of special education topics. This is an excellent source for parents who are learning to navigate through the Special Education System.

Resources for Families with Seriously Ill or Hospitalized Children

Fisher House

Members of the military and their families with loved ones who are hospitalized because of illness or injury must often travel far from home for specialized medical care. To help ease this difficult time, Fisher House Foundation donates "comfort homes," which are built on the grounds of major military and VA medical centers. There is at least one Fisher House at every major military medical center providing families in need with the comforts of home in a supportive environment. The average cost of staying at a Fisher House

en and their families in the hospital and their homes, arrange spe-
ations, and conduct fund-raising events for individual children. For
rmation, go to www.dreamfactoryinc.com or call 1-800-456-7556.

the World Village

s the World Village is a nonprofit resort that creates magical memo-
ildren with life-threatening illnesses and their families. Wish-grant-
izations coordinate transportation to Orlando, while Give Kids the
ovides accommodations at its whimsical resort, donated attractions
d meals for a week-long fantasy vacation. For more information, go
ktw.org or call 1-800-995-KIDS(5437).

LONG-TERM CARE

m care is care that you need if you can no longer perform everyday
ctivities of daily living (ADLs; see box below)——by yourself due
nic illness, injury, disability or the aging process. Long-term care
udes the supervision you might need due to a severe cognitive im-
t (such as a traumatic brain injury).

type of care isn't intended to cure you. It is chronic care that you
eed for the rest of your life. You can receive long-term care in your
me, a nursing home, or another long-term care facility, such as an as-
ving facility.

le often confuse long-term care with disability or short-term medical
ng-term care **is not**:

re that you receive in the hospital or your doctor's office
re you need to get well from a sickness or an injury
ort-term rehabilitation from an accident

rly 41percent of long-term care is provided to people under age 65 who
elp taking care of themselves due to diseases, disabling chronic condi-
injury, developmental disabilities, and severe mental illness.

al Resources

al Long-Term Care Insurance Program

ederal Long-Term Care Insurance Program (FLTCIP) is designed to
r your needs should you become disabled by an injury, illness, or aging.

is less than $10 a day, and many locations (
information, go to www.fisherhouse.org or (

Make-a-Wish Foundation

The mission of the Make-A-Wish Foundation
dren between the ages of 2 ½ and 18 with life-
Children must be referred to the foundation a
eligible for a wish by their physician. All wis
and family income is not a consideration in a
eligible to receive a wish. Contact Make-A-V
1-800-722-WISH(9474).

Starlight Starbright Children's Foundation

Starlight Starbright Children's Foundation is a no
to making a world of difference for seriously il
Starlight Starbright softens the hard edges of what
child has a serious illness. They work hard to meet
playrooms and teen lounges in hospitals and provid
so kids can play games, e-mail, chat with friends, a
from their hospital bed. They bring in entertainers
who are in the hospital. When the kids get to go hon
keep them connected through online chat rooms and
family. For more information, go to www.starlight.o

A Special Wish Foundation

A Special Wish Foundation, Inc. is a nonprofit cha
cated to granting the wishes of children who have be
threatening disorder. A Special Wish Foundation is tl
ing organization in the United States that grants wis
children, and adolescents from birth through and inclu
For more information, go to www.spwish.org or call

The Dream Factory

The Dream Factory, Inc., began with an idea to creat
tion dedicated to granting the dreams of children witl
nesses. Currently, there are more than thirty chapters a
with more than 5,000 volunteers who work to produc

visit child
cial celeb
more info

Give Kid

Give Kid
ries for c
ing orga
World p
tickets, a
to www

Long-te
tasks—
to a ch
also inc
pairme
This
might
own ho
sisted
Peop
care. L

- c
- c
- s

Ne
need
tions,

Fede

Fede

The
pay

ACTIVITIES OF DAILY LIVING (ADLS):

- bathing
  - o getting into a tub or shower
  - o getting out of a tub or shower
  - o washing your body in a tub, shower, or by sponge bath
  - o washing your hair in a tub, shower, or sink
  - o (If you need substantial assistance from another person to complete any one of these activities, you are dependent for bathing.)
- dressing
  - o putting on any necessary item of clothing (including undergarments) and any necessary braces, fasteners, or artificial limbs
  - o taking off any necessary item of clothing (including undergarments) and any necessary braces, fasteners, or artificial limbs
  - o (If you need substantial assistance from another person to complete any one of these activities, you are dependent for dressing.)
- transferring
  - o getting into a bed, chair, or wheelchair
  - o getting out of a bed, chair, or wheelchair
  - o (If you need substantial assistance from another person to complete any one of these activities, you are dependent for transferring.)
- toileting
  - o getting to and from the toilet
  - o getting on and off the toilet
  - o performing associated personal hygiene
  - o (If you need substantial assistance from another person to complete any one of these activities, you are dependent for toileting.)
- continence
  - o maintaining control of bowel and bladder function
  - o when unable to maintain control of bowel or bladder function, performing associated personal hygiene (including caring for catheter or colostomy bag)
  - o (If you cannot maintain control of bowel or bladder function and in addition you need substantial assistance from another person to perform the associated personal hygiene, you are dependent for continence.)
- eating
  - o feeding yourself by getting food into your mouth from a container (such as a plate or cup), including use of utensils when appropriate (such as a spoon or fork)

o when unable to feed yourself from a container, feeding yourself by a
    feeding tube or intravenously
o (If you need substantial assistance from another person to complete
    any one of these activities, you are dependent for eating.)

This insurance makes payments toward many types of long-term care including, but not limited to:

Nursing home care
Assisted living facility care
Formal and informal care in your home
Hospice care
Respite care

Employees, their spouses, adult children, employee's parents, and in-law
parents may be eligible to apply for this insurance program. Thanks to nego-
tiations by OPM (Office of Personnel Management) and the enormous buying
power of a group as large as the Federal Family, you'll find the premiums
very competitive and the coverage among the most comprehensive available
at any price. Your premiums can change only with OPM's approval and only
on a group basis. There is no government contribution for this program; you
will pay 100 percent of the premium.

Medicaid

Medicaid is a federal program administered by the states. Medicaid covers
basic health- and long-term care services for individuals with disabilities and
the elderly in families with low income and limited resources.
   *Note: Although Medicaid is intended to serve individuals with low income,
the program also serves others above the income limits.*
   Services and Benefits.   Those eligible for Medicaid benefits are entitled
to the following services, unless waived under section 1115 of the Medicaid
Law.

• Services for categorically needy eligibility groups:
   o Inpatient hospital (excluding inpatient services at institutions for men-
      tal disease)
   o Outpatient hospital including Federally Qualified Health Centers
      (FQHCs) and if permitted under state law, rural health care and other

ambulatory services provided by a rural health clinic which are otherwise included under states' plans

o Nursing facility services for beneficiaries age 21 and older

o Home health services for beneficiaries who are entitled to nursing facility services under the state's Medicaid plan

o Intermittent or part-time nursing services provided by home health agency or by a registered nurse when there is no home health agency in the area

o Home health aides

o Medical supplies and appliances for use in the home

o Physician services

o Laboratory and X-ray services

o Early and periodic screening, diagnosis, and treatment (EPSDT) for children under 21 (Under the EPSDT program, states are required to provide all medically necessary services. This includes services that would otherwise be optional services.)

o Family-planning services and supplies

o Medical and surgical services of a dentist

o Certified pediatric and family nurse practitioners (when licensed to practice under state law)

o Pregnancy-related services and service for other conditions that might complicate pregnancy

o Nurse midwife services

o 60 days postpartum pregnancy-related services

• Services for medically needy eligibility groups:

o Prenatal and delivery services.

o Postpartum pregnancy-related services for beneficiaries under age 18 and who are entitled to institutional and ambulatory services defined in a state's plan.

o Home health services to beneficiaries who are entitled to receive nursing facility services under the state's Medicaid plan

States may include any other services described under Medicaid law subject to any limits based on comparability of services. States may provide different services to different groups of medically needy. For example, states may opt to provide specific services for beneficiaries under age 21 and/or over age 65 in institutions for mental disease and/or intermediate care facilities for the mentally retarded, if included as medically needy. However, unless there is a waiver, the services provided to a particular group must be available to everyone within that group.

Family Support Services

Military families through the military family centers have access to a wide range of family support services, which typically include:

- Mobility/deployment assistance
- Information and referral
- Relocation assistance
- Personal financial management
- Employment assistance
- Family life education
- Crisis assistance

Centers may also provide:

- Individual, marriage, and family counseling
- Transition assistance
- Services to exceptional family members

Local Community Support and Help

The one thing to always remember is that you are never alone. Within the military there is an awesome network of support and in the local community you will find even more. Local churches can provide support, comfort, and counseling. There are local branches of the American Legion and American Red Cross and many other groups and organizations ready and willing to give help. Consult the Web and the local telephone directory to locate groups that can be of specific help. For instance if your child has cerebral palsy, contact the local chapter of United Cerebral Palsy.

Local Respite

Respite care provides temporary relief for families and caregivers by giving them time to engage in daily activities, thus decreasing their feelings of isolation; providing the family with rest and relaxation; improving the family's ability to cope with daily responsibilities; maintaining a family's stability during a crisis situation; helping preserve the family unit; and making it possible for individuals with disabilities to establish individual identities and enrich their growth and development.

Most respite care programs offer services to families on a sliding fee scale with hourly and/or daily rates. Respite care services can range from a few hours of care up to 3 months of care, depending on the needs of the families and the type of respite care program available in a community. The ages served by respite programs range from infancy to adulthood. Often programs serve a particular disability.

Respite care is provided at in-home or out-of-home settings. Many families prefer in-home respite care. There are several advantages to in-home respite care:

- The family member is comfortable in the home setting and does not have to adjust to different environments.
- The caregivers are often more comfortable if the family member does not have to leave the home.
- The home is already equipped for any special needs the family member may have.

Out-of-home respite provides an opportunity for family members with disabilities to be outside the homes with other children and adults.

Your family may benefit from respite care services. Ask yourself the following questions:

- Is finding temporary care for your family member difficult?
- Does caring for your family member sometimes interfere with scheduling appointments for yourself or your family?
- Are there projects around your home that you have not been able to complete because of the time required to care for your family member's special needs?
- Are you concerned that in the event of a family emergency there is no one you would trust to care for your family member?
- Would you be comfortable going to a trained and reputable respite provider to arrange for care for your family member?
- Do you avoid going out because you feel you are imposing on the family and friends who care for your family member?

If you answered "yes" to any of these questions, you and your family could benefit from respite care and should investigate the resources on your installation and in the civilian community.

Military Services Respite Care Programs

Army EFMP Respite Care Program

Eligibility for the Army's Respite Care Program is based on EFMP enrollment status, the exceptional family member's medical or educational condition and deployment needs. Families can receive up to 40 hours of respite per month for **each** certified exceptional family member. Read the revised Army Memorandum "Guidelines for Use of FY 07 Global War on Terrorism (GWOT) Funds for Exceptional Family Member Program Respite Care," dated 4 June 2007. Visit the MilitaryINSTALLATIONS directory to locate your local EFMP Manager.

Marine Corps EFMP Respite Care Program

The Marine Corps EFMP Respite Care is a program that provides temporary rest periods for family members responsible for the regular care of persons with disabilities. The Marine Corps EFMP Respite Care program provides up to 40 hours of respite care monthly for EFMP enrolled families. Respite Care may be provided by the installation CDC, FCC Home, Visiting Nursing Service, Family Member, or Neighbor. Interested families should contact their local installation EFMP Coordinator.

TRICARE's Extended Care Health Option (ECHO) Respite Care

On 1 September 2005, TRICARE's Extended Care Health Option (ECHO) replaced TRICARE's Program for Persons with Disabilities (PFPWD). The ECHO program has a new respite care benefit. It provides short-term care for a patient in order to relieve those who have been caring for him/her at home, usually the family. A maximum of 16 hours of respite care may be provided per month for any month a family member is receiving ECHO benefits. However, unused hours may not be banked for future use. This benefit is not meant to be a relief for parents to be deployed, be employed, seek employment, or pursue education. ECHO respite care services are provided by TRICARE–authorized home health agencies.

Military Child Development Programs

Although the military child development programs are not required to provide respite care for military families with special needs, families should register with the Children and Youth Office for assistance in locating an appropriate source of care. The cost would vary based on the hourly care rate at each installation, and parents would be responsible for paying for care.

Information on Respite Care

Many agencies and organizations have information on respite care services. These include but are not limited to your installation Community Services;

ARCH National Resource Center for Respite and Crisis Care Services; The Arc; and Parent Training and Information Centers.

The United Cerebral Palsy Association suggests that additional support can come through a respitality program, which offers a well-deserved break to parents from the constant challenges of child care. The respitality program combines respite services with quality hospitality services. Families benefit from the generosity of hotels and restaurants that provide free accommodations and a meal for two during a 24-hour getaway. This "mini-vacation" weekend can mean so much to families——it allows them to rejuvenate and refresh themselves so that they may return to their families with a brighter outlook.

Not all local UCP affiliates offer respite care or respitality programs. Please contact your local UCP to see if they offer individual and/or family supports groups, respite care, or respitality programs.

You should ask yourself the following questions when seeking respite care:

- What kinds of respite care will you need? (Short-term, long-term, or both, and why?)
- Do you prefer services provided in your home?
- Can you donate your time to a cooperative?
- Does the respite care agency provide the types of service you need?
- Is there a cost for the service?
- Who is responsible for direct payment to the provider?
- If you can't afford the service are there funds available to assist you? (Ask the agency.)
- How are the respite care providers selected?
- Are the providers trained?
- How many hours of training have they received?
- Were there criminal background checks completed during hiring?
- Are they trained in CPR/First Aid?
- What other areas of training have they completed?
- For out-of-home facilities, does anyone monitor the facility for safety and health measures?
- Will you be able to have a meeting with the provider prior to securing services?
- Can you provide written instructions for the providers?
- Can you assist in training the care provider with reference to your family member's needs?
- Will you have to carry additional home insurance coverage while the provider is in your home?

- Is there a policy for filing grievances or complaints? (If so, ask for a copy of the policy.)
- Can you request a specific provider and have that same person care for your family member each time?
- Will the provider care for your child's siblings too?

Medical Care: Caregivers, Child Care, Long-Term Care, Respite Care

- **Caregivers**
  - o National Family Caregivers Association——NFCA is a grassroots organization created to educate, support, empower, and speak up for the millions of Americans who care for chronically ill, aged, or disabled loved ones.
- **Child Care**
  - o NACCRRA, The Nation's Network of Child Care Resource and Referral—NACCRRA is the national network of more than 850 child care resource and referral centers (CCR&Rs) located in every state and most communities across the United States. CCR&R centers help families, child care providers, and communities find, provide, and plan for affordable, quality child care.
  - o Additional Child Care Resources——Resources for Child Care Outside the Home.
  - o Child Care Aware——Child Care Aware is a nonprofit initiative committed to helping parents find the best information on locating quality child care and child care resources in their community.
  - o Child Care Resource for Disasters and Emergencies——This site includes a wide range of information and resources about emergency preparedness, disaster and emergency response efforts, recovery resources, and lessons learned.
  - o Child Care Bureau/Bulletin—Inclusive Child Care-Quality Child Care for All since its creation in 1995, the Child Care Bureau has had a strong commitment to inclusive child care and has focused attention and resources on expanding and improving inclusive child care services throughout the country.
  - o Easter Seals—Easter Seals offers child care for children aged 6 months to 5 years.
  - o Joint Military Services and Boys and Girls Clubs of America Partnership—Mission Outreach_is an opportunity for children of Guard, Reserve, and Active Duty families to attend off-installation Boys and Girls Clubs free of charge.
  - o National Child Care Information and Technical Assistance Center—A service of the Child Care Bureau, this is a national clearinghouse and

technical assistance (TA) center that provides comprehensive child care information resources and TA services to Child Care and Development Fund (CCDF) administrators and other key stakeholders.

o National Network for Child Care/Special Needs—Provides a number of articles for child care providers on issues related to special needs children, for example, caring for children with challenging behaviors.

- **Long-Term Care**
  o Centers for Medicaid and Medicare Services—Information about Medicare long-term care.
  o National Long-Term Care Ombudsman Resource Center—Long-term care ombudsmen are advocates for residents of nursing homes, board and care homes, assisted living facilities, and similar adult care facilities. Long-term care ombudsmen advocate on behalf of individuals and groups of residents and work to effect systems changes. They provide an ongoing presence in long-term care facilities, monitoring care and conditions and providing a voice for those who are unable to speak for themselves. Find the ombudsman in your location through this site.

- **Respite Care**
  o Army GWOT-Funded Respite Care Program—Army guidelines for the Global War on Terrorism–funded Respite Care Program for qualifying soldiers enrolled in the Exceptional Family Member Program.
  o Air Force Aid Society Respite Care—A respite program for active duty Air Force families referred to the Air Force Aid Society by the Air Force Family Advocacy Program or Exceptional Family Member Program. The program is based on financial need.
  o Easter Seals—Easter Seals offers summer camps and respite care weekends.
  o TRICARE's Extended Care Health Option—An overview of the ECHO program, eligibility and coverage, cost shares, and other requirements.
  o The Arc answers questions on respite care—This is a good overview of respite care and how to look for a caregiver.
  o Arch National Respite Care Network—The mission of the ARCH National Respite Network and Resource Center is to assist and promote the development of quality respite and crisis care programs; to help families locate respite and crisis care services in their communities; and to serve as a strong voice for respite in all forums.
  o Armed Services YMCA Respite Care Program—The Department of Defense (DoD) has now authorized YMCAs in all fifty states as loca-

tions for implementation of this program. A list of licensed YMCA child care centers that are eligible to participate may be found on the YMCA website.

- Therapeutic Recreation
  - o The American Therapeutic Recreation Association (ATRA) defines "therapeutic recreation" as "the provision of Treatment Services and the provision of Recreation Services to persons with illnesses or disabling conditions. These services provide recreation resources and opportunities to improve health and well-being. Therapeutic recreation is provided by professionals who are trained and certified, and registered and/or licensed to provide therapeutic recreation to improve functioning and independence as well as reduce or eliminate the effects of illness or disability.
- Camps
  - o Summer programs provide unique opportunities for the development of social skills and interests that may get little attention during the school year where the focus is on cognitive learning. The recreational, social, and craft-oriented activities of a camp program may enhance a child's sense of self and develop his or her ability to get along with other children.

Additional Resources

Visit the MilitaryHOMEFRONT Resources section for Recreational Resources for Special Needs Individuals.

More Community Support

- American Legion—The American Legion is a large nonprofit veteran service organization that, with their fifty-five state organizations and 15,000 American Legion posts worldwide, have committed to support the needs of military personnel who are severely injured as they prepare to return to local communities.
- American Red Cross—Local chapters provide counseling, comfort items, and other disaster support. Also provide emergency communications services.
- AMVETS—Provides general assistance and advocacy, scholarships, career assistance, and phone cards through the National Program Department.
- Armed Forces Foundation—From referrals by family and friends, they provide emergency financial assistance, vehicle modifications, laptops,

housing assistance, tickets to recreation events, phone cards, and transportation assistance.

- Armed Services YMCA—Tuition assistance, counseling, recreation programs for youth and adults, child care, parent education, hospital assistance, health and wellness services, and respite care.
- Army Emergency Relief—Scholarships, emergency transportation and vehicle repair, and help with emergency financial needs for food, rent or utilities, medical, dental, and funeral expenses.
- Association of the United States Army—General advocacy and support with local chapters assistance with community support initiatives.
- Blinded Veterans Association—Counsels and links blind veterans with services and provides scholarships to family members of legally blind vets.
- Blue Star Mothers of America, Inc.—Provides air conditioners in summer and heat in winter and care packages and letters for troops.
- Boys and Girls Clubs of America—3,400 youth centers providing low-cost supervised after school and other programs for children 6–18 years old. Also scholarships and local community support programs.
- BPO Elks of the USA—Scholarships, youth programs, and grants to state Elks' organizations to improve the quality of life in their communities.
- Coalition to Salute America's Heroes—Emergency financial assistance, housing assistance, counseling, and employment assistance.
- Disabled American Veterans—Provides assistance with transition, homelessness, disaster relief grants for natural disasters, and other emergencies and general assistance and advocacy.
- DRS Technologies Inc.—The DRS Technologies Charitable Foundation supports Operation Mend, a partnership between Ronald Reagan UCLA Medical Center and Brooke Army Medical Center, San Antonio, Texas, to help treat wounded warriors. www.drsfoundation.net
- Fisher House Foundation—Provides airline tickets using donated frequent flier miles to military and family and friends who are hospitalized as a result of their service in OEF/OIF. Also provides temporary lodging and transportation support.
- Freedom Alliance—Scholarships, clothing, gift certificates, phone cards.
- Gold Star Wives of America, Inc.—General assistance provided by members whose spouses have died while serving on active duty.
- Granting Freedom—Provides home modification grants to severely injured service members who own or rent homes in Virginia.
- Helmets to Hardhats—Their Wounded Warrior program is a new supplement to the National Helmets to Hardhats program. Its purpose is to as-

sist disabled veterans in their search for new careers outside the military. Through the Wounded Warrior program, disabled veterans have access to a construction career database that includes career opportunities such as project supervisors, job estimators, and so forth. The Wounded Warrior page offers veterans the ability to create an online resume and participate in an online community to learn more about the many opportunities that are available. The program is self-selecting, allowing the veteran to apply to the many available apprenticeships and Wounded Warrior positions. Since its inception in 2003, the Helmets to Hardhats program has a reputation for creating a link to the best careers in the construction industry. And now, with the addition of the Wounded Warrior site, it is also creating a link to the best careers that support the construction industry.

- Homes for Our Troops—Builds new or remodels existing homes for veterans who meet the VA guidelines for the Special Adapted Housing Grant.
- Hope Coming Ministries—Located in Simi Valley, Southern California, this organization provides counseling services, specializing in counseling couples and individuals. Helps returning veterans adjust back into their communities and helps find jobs, education opportunities, and more.
- Injured Marine Semper Fi Fund—Financial grants to injured Marines and Sailors and their families during the immediate crisis period.
- Marine Corps League—Information and advocacy.
- National Amputation Foundation—Home or hospital visits for peer counseling, recreation events, and adaptive equipment support.
- National Veterans Legal Services Program—Provides legal assistance.
- Navy League of the United States—Public outreach, transportation discounts, and scholarships.
- Navy Marine Corps Relief Society (NMCRS)—The society is committed to helping Navy and Marine Corps families find the resources they need to deal with the changes in their lives as a result of service during wartime. They have both nursing support and financial services available as part of their Combat Casualty Assistance (CCA) and Combat Related Assistance (CRA). These services are beyond routine society assistance and can be requested on behalf of a wounded Sailor or Marine. CCA/CRA financial services include help with family travel and living expenses while convalescing, home and vehicle adaptations, and educational assistance.
- NMCRS's Visiting Nurse Combat Casualty Assistance Program—This program is available to provide medical and emotional support, as well as resource information on medical and resource information that may concern wounded Sailors and Marines and their entire family. A team of

visiting nurses provide long-term follow-up at major Navy and Marine Corp communities throughout the world.

- Navy Wives Clubs of America, Inc.—Scholarships, thrift shops.
- NetPets.org—MilitaryPetsFOSTER Project is a nationwide and global network of individual foster homes that will house, nurture, and care for the dogs, cats, birds, horses, and all other pets for all military personnel.
- Our Military Kids—Awards grants to children of severely injured Guard and Reserves for after-school programs.
- Rebuilding Together—The nation's leading nonprofit working to preserve affordable homeownership and revitalize communities.
- Serving Those Who Serve—Volunteer-based home rehabilitation organization, which provides no-cost services to severely injured service personnel who own their homes.
- Special Operations Warrior Foundation—Scholarships.
- United Spinal Association—Home modification grants, adaptive recreation programs, advocacy, and benefits support.
- Unmet Needs—VFW Foundation—Assistance with airfare, travel and lodging, child care, clothing, mortgage and rent, home and auto repair, and medical deductibles.
- USA Cares—Supports all military members and their families with grants for quality of life issues caused by military service. In partnership with the Homeowners Preservation Foundation, they have also saved hundreds of military homes from foreclosure. In partnership with Veterans Airlift Command, USA Cares coordinates transportation for injured Service members.
- USO—Scholarships, entertainment, and other morale support programs.
- Veterans Assistance Foundation—Referrals for psychological counseling, transitional assistance for homeless and housing assistance, and employment assistance.
- VFW—Public outreach, youth education, and other community support. Emergency financial assistance—one-time grants up to $500, relocation and employment assistance.
- Yellow Ribbon America—The National Guard Association of California: Organizes community outreach efforts to support their local deployed military members and families. Coordinates with local businesses, residents, churches, and community groups to focus resources. Their "Home Improvements for Our Troops" project is organizing communities to fund-raise to help make the necessary home improvements for injured veterans. Also helps communities organize "Welcome Home Celebrations."

County Support

Contact your local council for help in many ways. They can advise you on how to obtain disabled car placards, offer relief with paying bills in cases of hardship, perhaps provide child care and other support, and point you to other organizations that are able to assist you.

Many counties also offer their own therapy programs, in-home support, and respite care programs.

State Support

Again there are a wide range of services available through your state government, including family support programs, special education programs, and so on. Many states also have Heroes to Hometowns Committees, which act as a link among the Military Services and Veterans Affairs case workers at the military and VA hospitals, the severely injured member, their families, and their local community. Support has included:

- help with paying the bills
- finding suitable homes and adapting as needed
- adapting vehicles
- transportation to medical appointments
- finding jobs and providing educational assistance
- child care support
- arranging welcome home celebrations
- help working through bureaucracy and obtaining government benefits and entitlements
- sports and recreation opportunities
- holiday dinners

For more information go to www.legio.org/heroes.

FEDERAL SUPPORT

Make sure you are aware of and take advantage of all federal funding available to you.

TITLE V—Children with Special Health Care Needs (CSHCN)

Every state and the District of Columbia has a Title V program for Children with Special Health Care Needs (CSHCN) that is funded, in part, through the

Federal Title V Maternal and Child Health Block Grant and provides health and support services to children with special needs and their families.

As a result of the expansion of the eligibility criteria of state CCS programs, more and more children with chronic illnesses, developmental disabilities, sensory impairments, and other special health needs were being served. In recognition of this expanding responsibility and in response to criticism that the term "crippled children" was stigmatizing, Congress changed the name of this program in the Title V statute to State Programs for Children with Special Health Care Needs (CSHCN). In response to this change in federal legislation all states' Title V programs have deleted the phrase "crippled children" from their name. However, because the legislation did not mandate that states use a specific name, Title V CSHCN programs are known by different names in different states. Names given to CSHCN programs include: "Children's Medical Services," "Children's Special Healthcare Services," "Child Health Specialty Clinics," and "Division of Specialized Care for Children."

The federal Title V legislation also gives states the flexibility to use their Title V funds to design and implement direct care programs and services that are responsive to the specific needs of CSHCN and their families in the state, and accommodate the strengths and limits of the child health infrastructure in the state. Therefore, state Title V CSHCN programs have different financial eligibility criteria, serve different populations of children and youth with special health care needs, and provide and/or fund different sets of health care and related services. This can be confusing for a family with a child with special health needs, when moving from one state to another.

In addition to providing direct, personal health care services to eligible children, state Title V programs also have a responsibility to improve the quality and responsiveness of the overall health care system for children with special health care needs. States were given this "systems development" responsibility in 1989, when Congress amended Title V of the Social Security Act, and required that state CSHCN programs "provide and promote family-centered, community-based, coordinated care (including care coordination services . . .) and to facilitate the development of community-based systems of services for such children and their families." The 1989 amendments also allowed state Title V programs to continue to use federal funding to provide rehabilitation services to children under the age of 16 who receive benefits through the SSI program.

Over the last ten years, the Maternal and Child Health Bureau, at the federal level, in partnership with state Title V CSHCN programs, family leaders, and other professional and advocacy organizations have focused a significant level of effort on defining, describing, and making family-centered, community-based care available to all CSHCN and their families.

Family-centered care is a process that focuses on ensuring that:

- the organization and delivery of health-care services meet the emotional, social, and developmental needs of children.
- the families of CSHCN are integrated into all aspects of the health-care plan.
- families have alternatives and choices based on their own needs and strengths and receive support for those choices.
- the health-care system facilitates family/professional collaboration at all levels, especially in planning, implementing, and evaluating programs and their related policies and practices.

To accomplish this, state Title V CSHCN programs have worked to develop meaningful partnerships with families and promote leadership by families. State programs also provide the training, guidance, and policies that create these partnerships within each community as it builds its systems and services. Thus, the activities of state Title V CSHCN programs are not limited to providing and paying for health care for eligible children. Rather, these programs also fund family-to-family support organizations and support families in their efforts to play an active role in the development of programs and policies that are of benefit to all children with special needs and their families.

Services, Benefits, and Eligibility

Programs for Children with Special Health Care Needs provide access to medical services and programs for identification, diagnosis, treatment, and rehabilitation of children under the age of 18 (21 years of age and older in some states, depending on the diagnosis and funding available) with physically handicapping or potentially handicapping conditions, chronic illnesses, developmental disabilities, or sensory impairments.

Benefits may include:

- Early identification of health or developmental problems;
- Screening and /or assessment of the child and family's concerns, priorities, and resources;
- Tracking or monitoring;
- Therapeutic intervention(s) including family education and support and resource identification, referral, and coordination.

A number of other federal programs provide financial assistance to families. Some are limited to families with low income regardless of disabilities, and others provide assistance to families with special needs regardless of income. Here we summarize federal government programs that provide financial assistance to individuals and families either directly by cash payments or indirectly through some other means:

- **Supplemental Security Income**. SSI is a cash assistance program intended to meet basic needs for food, clothing, and shelter for those who are aged, blind, or disabled. **NOTE:** SSI is perhaps one of the most important federal programs, because eligibility for SSI may also provide automatic eligibility for other federal programs such as Medicaid, Medicare premiums, food stamps, and so forth. Adult SSI recipients are also eligible for federally funded, state-administered educational, vocational rehabilitation, and job-training programs.
- **Social Security Disability Insurance**. Social Security Disability Insurance pays monthly benefits to people unable to work for a year or more because of a disability.
- **Women, Infants, and Children (WIC)**. WIC provides supplemental foods, health-care referrals, and nutrition education for low-income pregnant, breastfeeding, and non-breastfeeding postpartum women, and to infants and children (birth to 5 years of age) who are found to be at nutritional risk. Individuals need not be disabled. WIC Overseas is a similar program provided by the Department of Defense for individuals assigned overseas.
- **Food Stamps**. Food Stamps are coupons available to low-income families. The coupons can be used like cash at grocery stores and commissaries. Individuals need not be disabled.
- **Family Subsistence Supplemental Allowance**. FSSA is the Department of Defense entitlement that increases a member's Basic Allowance for Subsistence (BAS) by providing a supplemental food allowance for military families. It is intended to remove the member's household from eligibility for benefits under the Food Stamp Program. FSSA will be paid in an amount equal to the total dollars required to bring that member's household income to 130 percent of the federal poverty line.
- **Medicaid/Medicare**. Although neither Medicaid nor Medicare provides finances directly to a family, they do assist financially by covering medical costs that may not be covered in other ways.
- **Earned Income Credit**. The EIC is a special tax benefit for working people who earn low or moderate incomes. It has several important purposes: to reduce the tax burden on these workers, to supplement wages, and to make work more attractive than welfare. Workers who qualify for the EIC and file a federal tax return can get back some or all of the

federal income tax that was taken out of their pay during the year. They may also get extra cash back from the IRS. Even workers whose earnings are too small to have paid taxes can get the EIC. What's more, the EIC reduces any additional taxes workers may owe.

4

Education

Your child may have a disability you are already aware of, or perhaps you suspect your child has learning problems but are unsure of what to do next. Learning how to navigate the special education system can be difficult for any family, but for military families whose educational environments are constantly changing, it is an even greater challenge. For any child in a military family where homes, schools, and neighborhoods frequently change, parents are the constant factor. If your child does not receive an adequate education, you and your child will cope with the consequences for years to come. As you learn the system and interact with professionals, remember that you are the expert on your child and that no one else has a greater knowledge or interest in your child than you do.

Separating the child from his or her non-disabled peers should only occur when the nature of the disability is such that education in a regular classroom, even with supplementary aids, cannot be achieved satisfactorily.

Parents play a key role in decision making. "Congress finds the following: Almost thirty years of research and experience has demonstrated that the education of children with disabilities can be made more effective by . . . strengthening the role of parents and ensuring that families of such children have meaningful opportunities to participate in the education of their children at school and at home" (IDEA 2004 Finding).

Procedural safeguards must be in place to ensure that the rights of the child and the child's parents are protected and that there are clear steps to follow in the case of a dispute.

The purpose of the Individuals with Disabilities Education Act (IDEA) is to ensure that all children with disabilities have access to a free, appropriate public education (FAPE), to ensure the rights of children with disabilities and those of their parents are protected, and to ensure that teachers and parents have the tools they need to meet educational goals and to assess the effectiveness of educational efforts being made for the child.

EARLY INTERVENTION SERVICES: CHILDREN FROM BIRTH THROUGH 3 YEARS

States, territories, and the Department of Defense provide early intervention services to infants and toddlers from birth to age 3 who are developmentally delayed or at high risk for a developmental delay.

The Department of Defense uses the term "early intervention services" or the acronym "EIS" when referring to early intervention services for infants and toddlers with developmental delays.

The following services are available:

Identification and Screening: Child Find, a required program in every state, territory, and DoD system, is a system designed to identify children who might require EIS/Part C. Many communities conduct periodic screening clinics to help identify children who might need EIS/Part C. If you suspect your baby or toddler has a disability or a developmental delay, you or anyone helping your family can ask for a screening. A visit to your military hospital or a call to your local school system will help you find a place to go.

Temporary Service Coordinator: Once a baby or toddler has been referred for EIS/Part C, a temporary service coordinator is assigned. This individual is responsible for keeping you informed of all steps to evaluate and to find appropriate services for your child.

Evaluation by a Multiple-Disciplinary Team: Evaluation refers to all of the procedures used to determine your child's unique strengths and weaknesses. The evaluation includes various procedures: observations, test(s), interviews, and other means of gaining information about your child. Based on the screening results, the temporary service coordinator will plan with you the procedures to be used in the evaluation.

Eligibility: Following completion of the evaluation, you and members of the multidisciplinary team meet and decide whether your child and family are eligible to receive early intervention services. Eligibility for services is based on certain criteria or standards with which your child's evaluation results are compared. Eligibility is based on the information you provide and whether the tests given indicate that your child meets any one of the three criteria:

- The child has developmental delays in one or more of the following areas: cognitive development; physical development, which includes vision and hearing; communication development; social or emotional development; self-help or adaptive skills.
- The child has a record of a diagnosed physical or mental condition which has a high probability of resulting in delay of development.
- The child is regarded as being at high risk of having substantial delays in development if early intervention services are not provided. *This is an optional criterion, which not all states have adopted.* The Department of Defense has not adopted this criteria.

Note: The IDEA allows states and the Department of Defense to develop their own eligibility criteria for EIS.

Individualized Family Service Plan: If your baby or toddler is found eligible for early intervention services, you and a team will meet to write a plan for addressing the unique needs of your child and your family. The plan, called an Individualized Family Service Plan (IFSP), is a written document that includes goals and outcomes for the child and family. Also included is a written plan for making the transition to services for your child when he or she is no longer eligible for early intervention.

Who Pays?

Part C of the Individuals with Disabilities Education Act (IDEA) does not require that all services be provided at no cost to families. Several early intervention services, however, must be provided at no cost to the family. These include evaluations or assessments, the development of the IFSP, and service coordination for eligible children and their families.

State Part C Programs: Some early intervention programs provide services at no charge to families. Other early intervention programs charge families on a sliding fee scale. The law says that no family shall be denied needed services because they cannot afford them. If you encounter problems related to costs or availability of services, contact your service coordinator or your Health Benefits Advisor. They are responsible for informing you of various options for finding other services, or for helping you arrange for the payments. Early intervention services might be paid for under your TRICARE option, your private insurance, or by Medicaid. A careful reading of your insurance policies and a discussion with your Health Benefits Advisor will inform you about what is covered, authorization procedures, and the frequency of services allowed. There are limitations under TRICARE on the duration and frequency of services. One thing to remember is that you can say "no" to any service recommended, including one or more that you don't want to pay for.

Note: In 1997, Congress amended Part C to state that IDEA Part C is payer of last resort "for services that would have been paid for from another public or private funding source, including any medical program administered by the Secretary of Defense." Congress thus clarified that TRICARE "pays first" for services that are otherwise eligible for reimbursement by TRICARE. The publication "TRICARE and Part C Guide to Services" clarifies the services for which TRICARE will pay.

DoD Early Intervention Services: All DoD EIS are provided at no charge to the families through the military treatment facility's Educational and Developmental Intervention Services (EDIS).

Directory for DoD Dependent Schools and Educational and Developmental Intervention Services: The Military Medical Departments through their Educational and Developmental Intervention Services (EDIS) provide Early Intervention Services (EIS) and related services in OCONUS locations where the Department of Defense Dependents Schools (DoDDS) is responsible for educational services. The OCONUS Directory is intended to assist the medical and educational assignment coordinators to identify those military communities outside the continental United States (OCONUS) with pre-established programs or services for children with special needs.

Eligibility

Age—Child 0–5 years of age: In the DOD programs, eligibility ends on the third birthday.

Income—Not applicable. Family income does not determine eligibility, but some states may charge on a sliding scale for services.

Categories—Federal law (the Individuals with Disabilities Education Act) and U.S. Department of Education regulations allow the lead agencies to define eligibility for early intervention services.

State Eligibility Definitions—Each state's lead agencies may define developmental delay somewhat differently. The National Early Childhood Technical Assistance System has developed a listing by state of the eligibility criteria for early intervention services.

DoD Eligibility Definition—The DoD schools have a consistent definition of developmental delay in DoDI 1342.12, enclosure 2 (definitions, p. 15):

E2.1.18. Developmental Delay. A significant discrepancy in the actual functioning of an infant, toddler, or child, birth through age 5, when compared with the functioning of a non-disabled infant, toddler, or child of the same chronological age in any of the following areas: physical, cognitive, communication, social or emotional, and adaptive development as measured using standardized evaluation instruments and confirmed by clinical observation and judgment. A child classified with a developmental delay before the age of five may maintain that eligibility classification through the age 8.

Head Start and Sure Start

Head Start and Early Head Start are comprehensive child development programs that serve children from birth to age 5, pregnant women, and their families. They are child-focused programs and have the overall goal of increasing the school readiness of young children in low-income families.

Head Start Enrollment Eligibility

- **Age:** Birth through 5 years of age.
- **Disability:** Ten percent of enrollments are offered to children with disabilities, regardless of income.
- **Income:** In order for a family to enroll their child in a local Head Start program they must meet the income eligibility requirements of the program. Specifically, a family's income must be below the poverty line (see income guidelines) or the family must be receiving public assistance; that is, SSI benefits. Note however that:
  Children who come from families with slightly higher income may be able to participate in Head Start when space is available. Your local program can discuss this with you.

For further information on eligibility, contact your local Head Start program.

Sure Start

Sure Start is a Department of Defense Dependents Schools (DoDDS) Program. Sure Start was established as a model school readiness program for families living and working at military installations overseas. Sure Start offers a comprehensive approach to early childhood education that involves children, their families, the school, and the community at large.

Sure Start is a preschool program that, like the Head Start model, is committed to providing the highest quality preschool education for eligible children of families living at military installations overseas. Like the Head Start model on which it is based, Sure Start is dedicated to providing comprehensive services in the areas of education, health, social services, and family involvement. Close collaboration between families, schools, and the community is seen as essential.

Sure Start Enrollment Eligibility

- **Military-connected:** Sure Start is a program for command-sponsored dependents.
- **Age:** It is primarily a program for qualified 4-year-olds. (The child must turn 4 years old by 31 October of the current school year.)
- **Family Dynamics:** Children qualify for Sure Start based on family dynamics that may put the child "at risk":
  o low income—based on rank (E-1–E-4)
  o single-parent household
  o parent(s) not a high school graduate
  o parent a teenager when first child was born
  o one or both parents speak a language other than English as their primary language;
  o low birth weight;
  o parent is on remote assignment (TDY) three months or more;
  o four or more children close in age, living in the home;
  o child has older sibling with a severe disability.

For additional information read DoDEA's publication "It Takes A Family; A Parent's Guide to the Sure Start Program."

SPECIAL EDUCATION: AGES 3 THROUGH 21

Special education is specially designed instruction, including physical education, which is provided at no cost to parents or guardians to meet the unique needs of a child with a disability (3 to 21 years old). Instruction might be conducted in a classroom, in the home, in hospitals or other institutions, and in other settings.

Special education involves a number of steps. In order to understand the special education process, you must understand these steps.

Referral: When a parent, school person, doctor, or friend notices that a child is not making progress at home or in school, that information is given in writing to the school system so that testing can take place to understand the child's disability.

Evaluation: An evaluation is a careful look by a team of teachers and specialists to determine a child's abilities, strengths, and weaknesses. Formal tests are given to gain information about the child's development in movement, communication, social relationships, behavior, independence and self-concept, senses/perception, thinking skills, and learning style. This information about the child's educational needs is used to determine whether a special education program is necessary.

Note: The term "Case Study Committee" is used in all DoD schools to denote the team of professionals and parents who make decisions about the special education program for an individual child. Public schools may use other terms for the school team.

Eligibility: In order for a child to receive special education, the child must first qualify according to established guidelines.

The Individuals with Disabilities Education Act (IDEA) defines disability categories, but each state and the DoD set the criteria. All states differ in their specific criteria. The Department of Defense schools in the United States and overseas use the same criteria, although the criteria may differ from that used in some states.

Individualized Education Program (IEP): Every child found eligible for special education must have an Individualized Education Program. The IEP is a written statement describing the specially designed program, including individualized goals and objectives, developed to meet the unique educational needs of the child. IDEA includes parents as members of the team to develop the IEP.

- The Department of Defense schools use a standard IEP form.
- Public school systems may use a variety of forms from state to state.

Placement: The placement decision identifies the appropriate school program and services needed to meet each child's educational goals. Program and services may include the classroom in which the child is placed, as well as support services such as speech therapy, occupational therapy, transportation, and other services needed by the child to assist in his or her learning. Again, parents are granted the right to participate in the placement deliberations and decisions.

Instruction: After the goals and objectives of the IEP are written, and a child has been placed in his or her school setting, learning activities begin in the classroom and in the support services. Parents and school personnel continue to work together to make the IEP and placement work for the child.

Annual Review: At least once a year the IEP is reviewed and a new IEP is developed for the next year.

Triennial Review: At least every 3 years, there is a review of the current data, evaluations if necessary, and an eligibility decision.

When the student turns 14: The school will include a statement of the transition services needed in the student's IEP. This statement, to be updated annually, should focus on how to plan the student's educational program through appropriate courses of study.

When the student turns 18: Under IDEA, beginning at least 1 year before students reach the age of majority under state law, their IEP must contain a statement that they have been informed of their rights under the law that will transfer to them as adults. The "age of majority" varies by state but generally occurs sometime between the ages of 18 and 21.

When the student turns 22 or graduates: Federal law requires that special education services must be available through age 21. Students with disabilities can use this time to acquire skills necessary for independent living or employment. These needs must be stated in the student's IEP and should include opportunities for community-based instruction and other adult objectives. However, some states interpret the law to stop education services at age 18 for special education students who graduate without receiving regular high school diploma.

CHILDREN OVER 21: GRADUATING/AGING OUT OF SPECIAL EDUCATION

When young adults with disabilities leave school, options for further educational and work opportunities differ among communities. The best way to determine the options in your community is to contact the local office of your State Vocational Rehabilitation Agency. Your local school director of special education may be able to provide parents and coordinators with information regarding postsecondary programs.

The following transition options may be available in your community:

- Competitive employment. This option covers regular jobs, paying at least minimum wage, in real work in integrated settings (full- or part-time jobs)
- Postsecondary education. This post–high school educational option includes learning that takes place in a college or university, community college, or vocational school or through an apprenticeship program.

- Transitional job training (TJT). TJT is a relatively short-term program (under 2 years) designed to provide those vocational services necessary to help an individual obtain employment in the competitive work world.
- Supported Employment. This option offers paid employment for persons with severe disabilities who need ongoing support to get and keep jobs. The goal of supported employment is to provide immediate opportunities for work and community participation while providing whatever level of support the person needs to participate in the workplace and the community. Initial on-the-job training is often provided by a job coach and supplemented by co-workers onsite.
- Sheltered Employment. Sheltered employment programs are not as prevalent as in the past. However, they do provide a work environment in a supervised setting. Sheltered employee productivity is supposed to equal at least 50 percent of an average worker. Workers are paid on a "piece rate" basis according to the number of items completed.
- Adult day programs. These programs take place in settings with other persons with disabilities. Depending on the individual, staff members assist clients in personal care, community living, and vocational skill development.

Choosing one or more of these options for your family member can help to ensure that he or she gets the skills necessary to a smooth transition from school to the workplace.

THE SPECIAL EDUCATION CYCLE

How does a child become involved in Special Education? When a child has an obvious or medically documented disability, or when a parent or teacher notices that a child is not progressing at the rate of his or her peers, this information is usually documented in writing within the school system. This type of referral begins the special education cycle. As the child moves through the cycle he or she will be assessed, and a decision will be made as to whether or not the child is eligible for special services. If deemed eligible, a unique Individual Education Program will be written and followed to ensure that the child will get an appropriate education.

Referral

A referral is simply a request, usually in writing, to have a child evaluated by the school system for special education services. Some school systems have a specific form for this. A referral for special education can be made by a parent, teacher, or doctor, or it can come from a child development program. This happens when someone involved with the child notices that the child is not making progress or showing signs of physical or behavioral challenges that are interfering with learning. Any of these people can contact the school system, in writing, and request that the child in question be evaluated. Usually, after a referral has been made, a screening committee meets to determine whether or not the child needs a full evaluation. This typically occurs at the child's home school. Should the screening committee decide that the child should have an evaluation, the parents will be notified as the child cannot be evaluated without their permission.

Evaluation

The evaluation is the series of tests and assessments the school system will use as they try to determine whether or not a child qualifies for special education.

A student's abilities may be evaluated in these areas:

Cognitive. A child's intellect (ability to reason, remember, and understand).

Behavioral. The ability to pay attention, the quality of the child's relationships with children and adults, and the behavior at home as well as school and other settings.

Physical. The assessment of the child's health to include vision, hearing, and the ability to communicate and move purposefully.

Developmental. The assessment of the child's progress in a number of areas such as understanding and responding to language, social and emotional levels, mobility, and ability to be organized.

You are an expert on your child, and the law requires that parents be included in every step of the evaluation process. It is important that you share your insight about your child. In fact, without your input, the school cannot have a complete picture of your child's personality and capabilities.

Sometimes talking to teachers and professionals about your child's areas of weakness may feel disloyal. However, without your perspective, the school system will not be able to fully understand your child and help him or her overcome or minimize areas of delay.

The school system must have a procedure that assures the following:

Parent(s) give written consent to testing before the child is evaluated.

Parent(s) give input about the child's growth and development.

The results of the evaluation will be available to parents.

Parents are given a chance to meet with representatives from the school so that parents can question any results they may disagree with.

Parents have an opportunity to examine the child's records.

The evaluation is appropriate for the child and without a cultural bias or not inappropriate because of the child's disability.

The assessment is given in the language the child is most comfortable with, unless this is not feasible.

Procedural Safeguards

Prior to 1 July 2005, state and federal regulations implementing the Individuals with Disabilities Education Act (IDEA) required school districts to provide the parent with a copy of procedural safeguards upon each notification of an Individualized Education Program (IEP) meeting. Since 1 July 2005, IDEA and state regulations implementing IDEA only require the provision of procedural safeguards statement to be given to the parent one time per school year. In addition to the once-a-year requirement, they must be given to a parent:

- Upon initial referral for evaluation;
- On the date the decision is made to make a removal that constitutes a disciplinary change of placement;
- Upon parental request for an additional copy;
- And, upon the first occurrence of the filing of a due process hearing request or child complaint, at which time the Department of Elementary and Secondary Education (DESE) provides the procedural safeguards statement.

Procedural Safeguards should be available both as a hard copy and online. They spell out the rights and obligations of both the parents and the education provider, definitions to avoid ambiguity, disciplinary measures, confidentiality clauses, complaints procedures, mediation and resolution, and so on.

Evaluation from the Child's Perspective

To many children, being evaluated is just another novel experience. The one-on-one attention can be fun. However, should your child feel anxious about the evaluation, spend some time talking about it. Explain that the evaluation is to help the child's teachers know the best way to help the child learn. On the day of the evaluation, be sure your child is well rested and fed. If you can, give your child a choice such as, "Which breakfast do you think will help you feel strong for your evaluation, oatmeal or eggs?" or "Would you like to wear your favorite shirt for your evaluation?"

When the evaluation is over, ask your child which activities were enjoyable and if there were things he or she didn't like. Praise your child for the effort.

Parents may or may not be able to observe or interact during the evaluation. However, if you think your child may be anxious or uncomfortable during the evaluation, even when working with an IEP assessment team to minimize challenges, then be sure to be nearby or in proximity. You are within your right to stop an evaluation if you feel that your child is not responding well to the experience, by showing signs of fear, agitation, or other extreme behaviors signaling problems.

The Evaluation Conference

The evaluation conference is when the findings of the formal evaluation will be discussed. This may be combined with the eligibility meeting. If you are not notified about such a meeting, you should request one. A copy of the evaluation report will be given to you.

What if There Is a Disagreement?

At this point, parents and the school system should agree that the evaluation results are accurate, complete, and up-to-date. If there is a disagreement, you can ask informally for more testing to be done. However, even informal requests should be followed up with an e-mail repeating your expectations. If this does not get the desired results, you can request an independent educational evaluation (IEE) of your child at public expense. You do not have to prove that the school's evaluation was faulty. You are entitled to an independent evaluation if there is reason to believe the initial evaluation incomplete or inaccurate. An IEE may evaluate any skill related to your child's educational needs. The school may not agree to this independent evaluation and may choose to hold a hearing during which they will try to show that the initial evaluation was valid and complete. Unless they do this, the school system cannot deny your request for a new evaluation. If, after a hearing the school system is not required to pay for an independent educational evaluation, you may still choose to have your child evaluated independently at your own expense. The school system is required to consider the independent evaluation when planning your child's education.

Should you agree with the school system that the evaluation is accurate, begin to discuss whether or not your child is eligible for special education. The Evaluation Conference may be held at the same time as the Eligibility Meeting.

Eligibility

Eligibility refers to the decision about whether or not a child qualifies for special education services based on the established criteria. A committee will make this decision. This committee is required to compare the results of the evaluation with the definitions of various disabilities as defined in the Individuals with Disabilities Education Act (IDEA). The following are the disabilities that qualify children who, because of their disability, require special education in order to benefit from their educational program:

Mental Retardation
Hearing, vision, speech, or language impairments
Emotional disturbance
Autism
Traumatic brain injury
Orthopedic impairments
Learning disabilities
Developmental delays for children between the ages of 3 and 9
Other health impairments

Each state, as well as the DoD, has its own categories and definitions of these disabilities. However, all states must follow the regulations under IDEA.

Eligibility Meeting

It is during this meeting that the decision will be made as to whether or not a child qualifies for special education. This meeting may be held at the same time as the evaluation conference.

Preparing for the Eligibility Meeting

One little-known and less-used technique is "Intent to record." You are within your legal right to record all IEP-related meetings. To do this, you will need to furnish the district with written notice of intent to record with ample notice for them to prepare to do the same. Typically you would also notify the district of any attendees, other than parents, such as advocates, who may also participate in a meeting. You will need to provide your own recorder. Digital recorders are fairly inexpensive and can record up to several hours of conversation if there is ample memory and space on the device. Recording every IEP meeting (from the beginning or when transitioning to a new district) is highly recommended because the recordings preserve the entire conversation and can be entered into evidence during due process if the district violates compliance with federal law. In many cases, recording IEPs is a simple step in making sure the meeting has the highest possible likelihood of being conducted in the appropriate manner by all parties. The district will also make their own recordings if you are known to also be recording the meeting.

Establishing an agenda and writing down any questions or talking points that you might have ahead of time will ensure that you cover all topics you intend to cover during the meeting.

Before the meeting starts you may want to pass around a picture or two of your child and family. This reinforces that your child is much more than an evaluation can measure. Be sure to ask for copies of the results of the evaluation as well as the official report of the meeting. Have your ideas about your child written down before going into the meeting. Include what you know about your child's way of learning and other information that may be helpful to the team. If desired, ask that your statement be included in the evaluation record. Be prepared to have specific medical evaluations or assessments from medical records that may strongly support your case for receiving special services and accommodations.

What if There Is a Disagreement?

If all goes well, you and the school system will agree on the best course of action for your child's education, be that in or out of special education. Problems may arise when you think your child qualifies and would benefit from special education services and the school does not, or if the school thinks special education appropriate, and you do not. Sometimes the problem may be that the school system and the parents of the child cannot agree on the nature or definition of the child's disability.

Should any of these disagreements occur, you may request an administrative review within the school system. If this is not available or if you are not satisfied with the results, there are two options. You may request mediation or a due process hearing, or you may request both at the same time. This will accelerate the process and lessen the amount of time your child must wait for an appropriate education.

Mediation is a process that allows a dispute to be resolved without litigation. When you mediate you have two goals: to resolve the dispute and to protect your relationship with the school system.

Due process hearings are conducted differently from state to state; however, they provide an opportunity to have your complaint heard in an impartial hearing. Before the hearing takes place, the school must hold a resolution session to give the parties a chance to resolve their differences before the hearing.

Consider hiring an advocate known to that school district. Many times schools will "reconsider" denials if they know you are prepared to invest the resources to enforce your child's legal rights.

Managing Emotions

As you walk into the meeting that is to determine whether or not your child will qualify for special education services, be aware of your emotions. You may be feeling worried, nervous, or even defensive. Try to put these feeling aside in this and subsequent meetings.

Focus on the goals you have for your child. Be a good listener, and let the others at the meeting know you understand their perspective. That does not have to mean you are agreeing with them.

If someone says something you don't understand, either about your child or the procedures used to qualify for special education, don't hesitate to ask. There is so much to absorb, and it can be overwhelming. If you still don't understand, ask again. While all parents want the best possible education for their children, it can be a blow to realize a child needs special education to grow academically. Bring your spouse, a friend, or a professional who knows your child with you. If your spouse is deployed, bringing someone with you to the meeting is even more important. This person can provide moral support as well as another perspective on your child. It is also nice to have someone with whom you can discuss the meeting.

Once the disagreements, if any, have been worked out, it is time to write your child's Individual Education Program.

Section 504 of the Rehabilitation Act

Section 504 is a civil rights law that prohibits discrimination on the basis of disability and applies to public schools among other entities. Because Section 504's definition of disability is broader than the IDEA's definition, some children who do not qualify for special education under IDEA do qualify under Section 504. This can be especially helpful for children with invisible conditions, such as learning disabilities or Attention Deficit Hyperactivity Disorder.

Individual Education Program (IEP)

An IEP is a written plan describing a detailed program for the child's education. It will contain the following:

  A description of the child's present level of academic achievement and functional performance.

Consideration of parental concerns about their child's education and progress.

Goals that are measurable and specific (e.g., David will write a paragraph with opening and closing sentences; or, Becky will feed herself with a spoon).

A list of the related services a child will receive and details about where the services will be located, who will offer them and for what length of time, and how much time the child will spend in the services.

Special Education Placement, which includes a description of how much of the day the student will spend in the regular education classroom with students who are not in special education, as well as a description of the special education programs and services that will be provided to the student.

The IEP will include the methods that will be used to determine if the child is meeting goals and objectives. This might be classroom observation, test results, or examples of school work.

The projected date for the beginning of services as well as the frequency, location, and duration of services.

Who Attends IEP Meetings?

The following people must attend the IEP meeting: the parent, a teacher of the child's regular education class (if the child is or will be in a regular classroom), a special education teacher, and an administrator who is not only knowledgeable about special education and the general curriculum, but is also able to commit the school's resources to meet the child's needs. Sometimes specialists and other educators attend. It may be appropriate for the child to attend, especially as parents begin to plan their child's transition out of school. Bring a spouse or friend to the meeting. It is a good idea to explain to this person the role they should take during the meeting (e.g., another viewpoint on the child or just moral support and another set of eyes and ears).

Preparing for the IEP Meeting

In order to prepare for this IEP meeting and future meetings, it is a good idea to take a little time to organize your child's school records. Many parents create an IEP notebook, which is kept up-to-date with copies of past evaluations, past IEPs, and correspondence with the school. If creating a notebook seems overwhelming right now, be sure to have a designated folder for all special education paperwork until you have time to create a notebook.

Potential Problems

You may be presented with an IEP that was completed before the meeting. Should this happen, keep in mind that you have the right to participate in the development of your child's IEP. Consider and refer to this IEP as a draft. If you feel pressured to sign it, simply remind the other members of the committee that you need time to read and digest such an important document, and that you will need a copy to take home with you. You have the right to have any draft IEP reviewed by an advocate. You do not have to sign an IEP you have not reviewed or have disagreement with. You can have your concerns or disagreement documented in the IEP as well.

If the school system says a course of action is prohibited by law or regulation, ask politely for help identifying this law or regulation.

FOCUS ON YOUR CHILD'S NEEDS

This is another time when emotions can run high because your child's education is so important. Remember to keep the needs of your child the focus of the discussion. When possible, have educational options for your child already in mind. If you feel resistance to your ideas, suggest trying a new idea for 8 weeks to see how it works. Look for common ground and be sure the others in the room know you are trying to understand their point of view. Remember that a pleasant attitude is much more productive than a negative one and thank those who have been helpful.

ARE YOU SATISFIED WITH THE IEP?

If you are satisfied with the IEP, sign it to show you accept the plan. If you would like a few days to think about it, you can ask for that. If you do not agree with all or part of the IEP, identify which parts are unacceptable. If the school refuses to make the changes, three options are available:

- Sign the IEP but indicate in writing the parts you find objectionable. You will then be on record as stating that you believe that the IEP does not meet all your child's needs.
- Sign the IEP but list the parts you find objectionable and write that you plan to appeal those parts. This way your child can begin or continue to receive the services while the appeal is pending.
- Refuse to sign the IEP and indicate in writing that you plan to appeal the IEP. Before doing this, ask what services your child can receive while

the appeal is pending since he or she may be denied services until the IEP is signed.

Remember, parental consent for an evaluation is not consent for a child to receive special education services. The school must have an informed consent before providing services.

Your child's IEP will be reviewed each year and rewritten to reflect the gains your child has made and the new goals that have been set. Because your input is crucial to the completeness of the IEP, the school system is required to notify you in writing when a meeting is scheduled. Once your child reaches the age of 16, the school is required to include him or her in meetings to address the transition from high school into post–high school life. If you would like to request the IEP team meet midyear to discuss your child's progress, you need to do so in writing.

Placement

Placement refers to the setting in which a child will be educated, including the school, classroom, and related services, and how much time the child will spend with children who are not disabled. The details of your child's placement should be spelled out in the IEP. An integral part of IDEA is the concept of the Least Restrictive Environment (LRE). This means that a child with disabilities should be removed from the regular classroom only when the child's disability is of a nature that it is necessary to do so.

Placement options.   School systems are required to provide a range of placement options to ensure differing needs can be met. This spectrum of placement starts with the general education classroom, moving to time in a resource room or "pull out" classes for certain subjects, to self-contained classrooms with only special education students, to private school, and finally to residential placements. Once you know which specific services your child will need, you can address the question of where these services should be provided. The focus is on how to best educate your child in the least restrictive environment. Least restrictive environment also means that whenever possible your child should be educated at the neighborhood school that he or she would normally attend, unless the IEP requires another arrangement. When appropriate placement cannot be provided by the public school system, a private day or residential school must be paid for at public expense.

Instruction and Related Services

Instruction is the actual educating of a child. It refers to time spent in the general education classroom and special education, as well as time receiving related services.

After all the evaluations and meetings have been held, the instructional time should be structured in such a way that your child's needs for an education are being met. Although the majority of instruction time is spent in school, parents have an important part to play as back-up for their child's teacher. It is up to you to create a homework routine that will work for your child and family and to help your child remain motivated and feel successful.

Remember that children learn best when they are relaxed. If your child is stressed about an assignment, he or she may not be able to do the work for worrying about how to get it done or fear of not doing well. Help your child by showing how to break the task into more manageable parts. Some teachers call this "chunking." The first step might be to read the directions, gather supplies, and then perhaps make an outline of what the child will do to complete the assignment.

If learning a new concept, be sure the child understands the vocabulary involved. Instead of asking, "Do you understand these words?" say, "Can you tell me what germination is?" A good place to start is to find out what the child already knows. Ask the child, "What can you tell me about George Washington?" Almost any answer can be used as a good beginning to start a conversation. Children will remember new information better if they can relate it to something they already know.

Writing can be especially challenging to a child who learns differently. To write, the child must do many things at once. First, the child must hold the story in his or her head, tell it in the correct order, remember punctuation and spelling, and once all this is done the child may feel defeated because the end result looks so messy. Brainstorm with your child before writing begins about words that might be used and have them listed near by.

Related Services

Your child's IEP may specify services other than those provided by the classroom teacher. The following are some of the related services your child may receive:

Assistive Technology. Any piece of equipment that improves a child's ability to communicate, to be independent, and to learn. It could be an augmentative communication board or a wheelchair.

Audiological. Services to identify children with hearing loss and to help with language improvement, speech, lipreading, conversation, or the appropriate use of hearing aids.

Counseling. School counselors who work to improve behavior, self-control, and self-esteem of students.

Medical. Available for diagnostic reasons and to make recommendations for specialized services based on the child's disability.

Occupational Therapy. Activities focus on fine motor skills, such as writing, sorting, eating, and other skills that assist in improving daily life.

Orientation and Mobility. Assistance for any child who needs to be taught how to travel around the school building, perhaps because of visual impairment.

Parent Counseling and Training. Helps parents of children with special needs to understand how their child is developing, and also refers to other groups who can offer financial planning or other professional services.

Physical Therapy. Provided by a licensed therapist, this service concentrates on gross motor functioning. That is, large body movements like sitting, standing, and moving.

Psychological. School psychologist gives testing, interprets results, and acts as a consultant to school staff.

Rehabilitative Counseling. Independence training, employment preparation, vocational training, and integration into the workplace.

School Health Services. Nursing services that are necessary to assist a child so he or she will benefit from the educational plan must be described in the IEP, and may be services such as administering medication, providing assistance with catheterization, or breathing therapy.

Social Work. Provides group or individual therapy and helps with problems in the child's home that may affect the child's adjustment in school.

Speech. Diagnoses speech and language disorders, provides therapy, and counsels parents and teachers regarding speech problems.

Transportation. Schools are responsible for transportation of special education students to and from school and in and around the building.

There may be other services that the IEP team identifies that are not on this list. Specific goals will be written for related services, just as goals are written for class work.

Finally, You Have a Plan

Now that you are past the evaluation stage and have a written plan and a comfortable routine, relax a little. You deserve it. It is a good idea to give your child's teachers a little time to get the program running smoothly before checking on it. Once the school year is underway and the teacher has had a chance to get your child's program up and running, establish an atmosphere of cooperation with the teacher. This is essential to keeping track of your child's academic, behavioral, and social activity in the classroom. Some parents and teachers stay in touch by way of a notebook that is passed back and forth every day, by telephone, or by frequent conferences. Probably some combination of the above is best. Be as positive as you can be and let the teacher know that you appreciate the work done on behalf of your child.

Annual Review

Once a year the school system is required to review your child's individual education program. This is called the annual review. Your school system is required to notify you in writing of the purpose of the meeting and who will attend. It should be attended by at least three people: the parent, the teacher, and a representative of the school system who is authorized to commit school resources. If your child spends time in a regular classroom, the teacher of that class must attend. In addition, specialists such as the school psychologist, an occupational therapist, or the school nurse may attend. The meeting must be at a time and place that is convenient for you. Also, if you need assistance with English, they must provide an interpreter.

There is an option in some states to replace the annual review with a review every 3 years. The benefit may be that teachers spend less time on paperwork this way. However, children grow and change a lot in 3 years, and if you are not comfortable with this idea you may opt for an annual review. As with the evaluation conference and the eligibility meeting, have your thoughts, ideas, and questions written down before the meeting begins. You may want to bring someone with you, a spouse or friend, who has seen your child progress.

Triennial Review

Every 3 years the school system is required to conduct an extensive review of your child's progress. This is called the triennial review. There may be entirely new evaluations done, and there will be a new eligibility decision about whether to continue special education. There will be a thorough review of existing data to determine which new evaluations may be needed. If there are any new areas of suspected disability, you may request certain evaluations, and unless they provide rationale for refusing, the school is required to provide them.

Records

Many school systems keep three types of records:

Cumulative File. This file contains report cards, standardized test scores, teacher reports, and a copy of your child's Individual Education Plan

(IEP) if your child is already in special education. You can get a copy of this through your school office.

Confidential File. This may be kept at the school or an administrative office. It has all the reports written about your child's evaluation, medical records if available, summaries of meetings held by the evaluation team, and sometimes a record of your correspondence with the school. Ask the principal to see this file.

Compliance File. Some school systems keep a separate file with all reports, records of meetings, and all correspondence. You can ask the principal if this file exists.

To receive copies of any of these files, ask your school system what the procedure is. If you request copies of your child's records, the school must provide them, but there may be a charge for the cost of copying. You must request a copy of your child's records in writing.

Transition to Adulthood

If your child has been involved with special education for several years, you have a good understanding of the IEP process. Transitioning out of school and into the world has a different focus. Instead of identifying and working to minimize your child's challenges, you are looking toward the future and exploring what it will take for your child to learn a job or live on his or her own.

Once a child graduates or leaves the school system, there is no guaranteed program to pick up where IDEA leaves off. However, starting between the ages of 14 and 16, your child's IEP will address the transition process. Transition services are a coordinated set of activities that will aid a child with a disability as he or she moves from school to post-school activities. These activities should be based on the child's needs, taking into account his or her strengths and interests.

Your child should be assisted in developing post-school living objectives concerning employment or daily living skills. Time in school might be spent with an emphasis on practical life matters, like reading job applications or menus and learning money skills. Ask your child what kind of work he or she would like to do. Is it realistic? Is there a compromise that can be made so that your child's desires can be met? Perhaps a child who wants to be a veterinarian could work in a vet's office.

These transition services should start no later than the first IEP in order to be in effect when the child turns 16, and should be updated annually thereafter. Also, no later than 1 year before reaching the age of majority under state law, your child must be informed of his or her rights under IDEA, if any, that will transfer to him or her upon reaching the age of majority.

What options are there for your child?

College. Whether two- or four-year, colleges offer opportunities for students with disabilities to continue their education. Because of the Americans with Disabilities Act (ADA), colleges cannot discriminate against otherwise qualified students with disabilities.

Continuing and Adult Education. These courses range from computer skills to cooking and offer a way to expand your child's horizons.

Vocational Training. There are trade schools that typically prepare students for specific occupations, such as beautician or electrician, and require a high school diploma to attend.

On-the-Job Training. Short-term training that allows a child to learn a job while working on the site. Many vocational rehabilitation agencies, disability organizations, and large companies provide this sort of training and placement.

Competitive Employment. These are jobs in the mainstream of everyday life. Competitive employment describes jobs for which your child would get paid the going rate. The law prohibits discrimination and requires reasonable accommodations be made if the person is qualified for the job.

Supported Employment. This is paid employment for people with severe disabilities, who have a job coach that provides guidance by helping the employee improve job skills or any other job-related needs. Generally the coach is involved heavily in the beginning of employment, but is less involved as the employee gains in skill and comfort.

Adult Day Programs. These programs provide a work environment in a supervised setting with other disabled workers. They will usually receive training in life skills and recreation.

Centers for Independent Living. Here people with disabilities develop self-help and advocacy skills like balancing a checkbook, cleaning, and cooking nutritious foods.

Guardianship and Declaration of Incapacitation

Usually when a child reaches the age of majority, 18 in most states, it is assumed that he or she will be able to make decisions about health, finances, and the future. However, for some children this not the case. Once your child reaches the age of majority you will have no control over educational, financial, or health-related decisions your child might make. If you are concerned that your child will not be capable of making these decisions responsibly, consider asking the courts for guardianship. The age of majority varies from state to state. Check www.militaryhomefront.dod.mil/efm to find out information about your state.

Guardianship is a court-approved relationship between a legal guardian and the person with a disability. The court will define the degree of legal authority that the guardian will have to act on behalf of the disabled person. Detailed documentation from a physician will be needed to show that your child is not mentally capable of becoming independent.

Laws concerning guardianship vary from state to state; so if you move to another state, you will have to reapply in the new state.

FEDERAL LAWS

Three federal laws provide the legal foundation for the education of children who have disabilities:

Individuals with Disabilities Education Improvement Act of 2004

In August 2006, the secretary of education, Margaret Spellings, announced the release of the Individuals with Disabilities Education Improvement Act of 2004. IDEA requires early intervention services for children from birth until 3 years of age with disabilities or developmental delays and special education for children with disabilities from 3 through 21.

Nondiscrimination Rehabilitation Act of 1973, Section 504/Regulations

Section 504 of the Rehabilitation Act prohibits discrimination against people with disabilities by any agency or organization that receives federal funds. Recipients of federal funds such as states, counties, cities, public and private schools, hospitals, and clinics must make it possible for people with disabilities to participate in their programs. However, Section 504 is not required overseas, and is limited to the United States and its territories. The regulations governing Section 504 call for a free, appropriate education for all children with disabilities, regardless of the nature or severity of their disability. Positive efforts to create job opportunities are required so that a disability is not a barrier to employment. College and other postsecondary education options are to be adapted to the needs of students with disabilities. People with disabilities must receive equal treatment by education, health, welfare, and social service agencies.

An agency can be penalized by loss of federal funding if it discriminates against a person with disabilities. Any person who feels discriminated against can notify the Office of Civil Rights (OCR). You can contact the regional office that serves the state in which the discrimination occurred. Ask the regional office for help in writing the complaint.

Both IDEA and Section 504 reinforce and strengthen each other. They both stress that young people with disabilities must have every possible opportunity to take part in the normal life of school, both in academic and extracurricular activities.

Since 1975, each state has passed special education laws and regulations that are consistent with IDEA. State laws provide guidelines that local school districts must follow as they make special education programs and services available to children with disabilities.

Americans with Disabilities Act (ADA)

Congress passed the Americans with Disabilities Act (ADA) in 1990. Like Section 504 of the Rehabilitation Act, ADA prohibits discrimination against students with disabilities. The ADA and Section 504 are described as nondiscrimination statutes rather than as entitlement statutes such as IDEA. They provide procedures to ensure that persons with disabilities enjoy the same rights as persons without disabilities. When those rights are thought to be violated, the ADA, like Section 504, provides a procedure for addressing the alleged violations.

ADA and Section 504 are used to benefit both those children with disabilities that require special education, as well as those children who have a disability but are not eligible for special education services. To qualify for protection under ADA and Section 504, your child must show that the disability "substantially limits" a major life activity, such as walking, seeing, hearing, speaking, learning, working, taking care of oneself, breathing, and performing manual tasks. Many children with these impairments are eligible for special education services under IDEA. Some children, however, will not qualify for special education, but if found eligible under Section 504 or ADA, they will qualify for equipment, aids, or other accommodations needed to help them benefit from the school program.

Because of the similarity and overlap of ADA and Section 504, the U.S. Department of Education generally uses Section 504 to interpret the ADA in educational issues.

IDEA (Individuals with Disabilities Act)

The Individuals with Disabilities Education Act (IDEA) is the special education legislation that guides school systems throughout the United States, its territories, and Department of Defense schools in the education of children with special needs. IDEA Part B establishes educational requirements for children with disabilities from the ages of 3 to 21. IDEA Part B has six major principles that must be met by school systems:

1. Free and Appropriate Public Education (FAPE). This means that your child is entitled to an education at public expense, under public supervision and direction.
2. Appropriate Evaluation. This includes gathering the information necessary to ensure a child is able to be involved and progress within the general curriculum of the school.
3. Individualized Education Program (IEP). This is a written plan for a child with a disability that is developed and reviewed according to the standards detailed in IDEA.
4. Least Restrictive Environment (LRE). Children with disabilities are most appropriately educated with non-disabled peers.
5. Parent and Student Participation in Decision Making.
6. Procedural Safeguards.

NON-DOD SCHOOLS PROGRAM

Families who will be serving in an overseas area where the DoD does not operate a school have a variety of options ranging from home-based schooling programs to private or public schools. The Non-DoD Schools Program (NDSP) provides support and funding for the education of authorized command-sponsored dependents of military members and DoD civilian employees assigned to overseas areas where no DoD Dependents School is available within the commuting area.

The NDSP-Americas is responsible for locations throughout Central and South Americas, Mexico, Canada, and the Caribbean Islands. Local NDSP liaisons have been established at all locations to assist sponsors with registration and to facilitate the funding process.

If you are expecting an assignment to a location throughout Central or South America, Mexico, Canada, or the Caribbean Islands, please contact the NDSP-Americas Program Manager for information on your local NDSP liaison.

Upon receiving assignment orders to an overseas location where there is no Department of Defense Dependents School (DoDDS), contact the local NDSP liaison at your gaining command/new location. The liaison will provide information on available schooling options at that location.

Parents may not make a commitment of U.S. Government funds to any educational institution without obtaining approval from the NDSP Program Manager.

Once you have gathered information about the educational options available and decide which option is best for your dependents, please contact your local Non-DoD Schools Program Liaison for the current enrollment procedures.

The following are the procedures that the Department of Defense Education Activity (DoDEA) follows in the identification and provision of special education services for eligible Department of Defense (DoD) dependents residing in areas where there is no DoDEA school. Prior to any special education activity, Non-DoD School Program (NDSP) entitlements and command sponsorship must be verified.

The DoDEA NDSP is committed to the provision of appropriate special education and related services for DoD dependents who are space-required and eligible for NDSP under DoD Directive 1342.13, "Eligibility Requirements for Education of Minor Dependents in Overseas Areas," 8 July 1982, as amended. It is the intent of the NDSP to follow the guidance and principles set forth in DoD Instruction 1342.12, "Provision of Early Intervention and Special Education Services to Eligible DoD Dependents," 16 December 2003; which is the DoDEA's implementing instruction for IDEA (Individuals with Disabilities Education Act).

If your child is having difficulty academically or socially in the overseas school, contact your liaison officer. The liaison will begin the collaborative decisions about what services are recommended by the school. If your child is referred to have a comprehensive diagnostic evaluation due to a suspected disability, the Area NDSP POC facilitates the required assessments and location. Your permission is needed prior to beginning any funded formalized assessments.

The purpose of the assessments is to provide insight into factors influencing your child's academic and or behavioral problems that are interfering with his or her educational success. If your child's school does not have the special education resources, the NDSP Special Education Eligibility allows the funding for extra services such as tutoring, counseling, and speech services.

Prior to incurring any expense, authorization of payment for the cost of any service must be issued by the NDSP. DoD sponsors assigned to overseas locations are not authorized to obligate the U.S. Government, contract with a private institution, or charge educational fees to DoDEA appropriations, that is, Foreign Military Sales, Security Assistance Office, or Military Assistance Program case funds, without obtaining prior approval from the DoDEA NDSP.

Prior to any funded educational services, command sponsorship must be verified.

Home-Based Educational Programs

The Non-DoD Schools Program (NDSP) provides support and funding for the education of eligible dependents of sponsors assigned at locations where the DoD does not operate a school within commuting distance.

Parents electing to provide home-based educational instruction rather than enrolling their child in a local school must proceed through the following steps:

- Select a home-study program.
- Submit the following documentation to your local NDSP liaison:
  - o A copy of the sponsor's orders plus any amendments.
  - o A copy of the sponsor's overseas tour extension approval if the DE-ROS (Date Estimated Return Overseas) has expired or will expire prior to the beginning of school. Documentation of a current DEROS is required for continued enrollment in the Non-DoD Schools Program.
  - o DoDEA Form 610, "Application for Enrollment in a non-DoD School," for each dependent. A new DoDEA Form 610 is required anytime there is a change in schools.
  - o "If the child(ren) is/are applying for entry to Kindergarten or First grade, we require a copy of that child's Passport or Birth Certificate to verify age if the PCS orders doesn't reflect the birth date or the birth date is incorrect on the orders. It is DoDEA policy that a child must reach 5 or 6 years old for entrance into kindergarten and first grade respectively. In the Northern Hemisphere where the school year starts in August, the child must reach 5 or 6 years old by September 1 of the enrolling year. In the Southern Hemisphere where the school year starts in January, the child must reach 5 or 6 years old by February 1 of the enrolling year."
  - o If the dependent's names are not listed on the sponsors' orders or in a separate approval authorization, a completed "Certification of Command-Sponsored DoD Dependents" form is required.

The maximum allowable school-year rate for home-based educational instruction is $5,700 for grades kindergarten through 8 and $7,700 for grades 9 through 12.

Reasonable materials may only be ordered for the current grade in which the dependent will be enrolled (grade/age appropriate basis). Materials may not be ordered for two academic years in one school year. Curriculum materials may be ordered for one grade level above or below the grade of enrollment in one curricular area only.

Allowable homeschooling expenses include:

1. Traditional curriculum textbooks and other supplemental materials as may be appropriate for math, science, language arts, social studies, and other subjects on a grade/age appropriate basis.
2. Instructional CDs/software, curriculum guides, and manipulative materials for math, etc.
3. Fees charged by local public or private schools for access to libraries, computer lab and group participation in athletic, extracurricular, or music activities that are normally free of charge in U.S. public schools.
4. Fees for curriculum-related online Internet services such as study programs, library services, and distance learning.
5. Rental of curriculum-related equipment such as microscopes or very large band instruments (such as a Sousaphone) that would normally be provided by U.S. public schools.
6. Required testing materials by either the formal home-study course or other authorized program.
7. Advisory teaching service affiliated with the selected formally recognized home-study course.
8. Tuition charges, shipping costs, lesson postage, online Internet and facsimile charges associated with formal recognized home-study course or other authorized program.

Nonallowable homeschooling expenses include:

1. Equipment such as computers, keyboards, printers, televisions, facsimile and scanning machines, calculators, microscopes, and furniture.
2. Non–course specific CDs, videos, DVDs.
3. General reading materials and reference materials (dictionaries, encyclopedias, globes) etc.,
4. Purchase or rental of items that have broader use than the course being studied (i.e., computer hardware, calculators, band instruments except as noted above).
5. Expendable supplies (paper, pencils, markers) that are normally purchased by parents in the United States.
6. Parental training in home-study private instruction.

7. Any form of compensation to the parent such as child care or supervisory costs.
8. Travel and transportation costs at post or away from post.
9. Personal telephone, Internet, satellite, cable, or other available communication subscription fees.
10. Fees for museums, cultural events, or performances that would normally be paid by parents in the United States.
11. Private lessons.
12. Membership in gymnasiums, cultural clubs, spas, and other private clubs.
13. Textbooks, Bibles, workbooks, daily devotionals, or any material primarily for religious instruction.
14. Insurance associated with shipping charges. (Do not elect the optional insurance.)
15. Fees to an independent agency for posting credits and issuing transcripts.

Documentation for Payment or Reimbursement

Sponsors who elect to purchase educational curriculum materials for home-schooling purposes must submit to the local NDSP liaison receipts and an itemized list indicating the appropriate dependent(s) for each purchase. Sponsors are responsible for out-of-pocket expenses until the purchase is approved and reimbursement processed. Responsibility for documentation rests with the sponsor. Receipts must be legible. Itemized lists of educational texts or materials must clearly indicate relevance to curriculum areas.

Supplemental Instructional Support

Tutoring/Correspondence Course/Second Language

Supplemental instructional support may be reimbursed up to the allowable rate but must be **pre-approved**. In addition to the Department of State Standardized Regulations (DSSR) educational allowance for a particular location, $3,000 per school year may be authorized only for the following reasons:

- The approved school does not provide instruction in academic subjects generally offered by public schools in the United States for students in grades 9–12 (i.e., English, United States history, United States government, geometry, algebra), and the student will have no other opportunity to complete the courses prior to graduation.

- The approved school offers its curriculum in a language that the child does not know well enough in order to progress in the curriculum.
  - o If the location does not have a tuition-free school with English language–based instruction, the next priority is a tuition-paying local school with English language–based instruction. If the parent elects to place the student in a local tuition-free school where the language of instruction is other than English, approval may be granted for tutoring in the other-than-English language of instruction on a case-by-case basis up to the maximum allowable rate for supplemental instructional support.
  - o When there is no school with English-language-based instruction and the parent must enroll the student in a local school where the language of instruction is other than English, approval may be granted for tutoring in the other-than-English language of instruction on a case-by-case basis up to the maximum allowable rate for supplemental instructional support.
  - o Authorized services are based on the language proficiency and age of the child.
- The approved school requires additional instruction to enable the child to enter a grade or remain in the same grade in the school.
- The child, upon returning to post along with his/her family subsequent to an authorized/ordered evacuation, requires additional instruction to successfully complete the current school year.
- The child requires assistance in basic classes:
  - o In grades K–3, the student requires compensatory/supported instruction because he/she is not progressing or performing within the normal developmental range.
  - o In grades 4–12, the student is failing or in jeopardy of failing.

The sponsor and school must submit documentation in evidence of the request. This may include current grade/progress reports and narrative description of current functioning from the teacher. Additional information may be requested. Approvals are generally for a 9-week period. Requests for extended tutoring must be accompanied by a progress report for the previous period of authorized assistance.

Tutoring time is based on the age of the child and the curricular areas being addressed. Tutoring is generally authorized for 1 to 5 hours per week. Tutoring will not be authorized to assist in completing homework.

Materials required for language instruction/tutoring must also be approved in advance.

Frequently Asked Questions

Q. What is the "NDSP"?

A. The "NDSP" stands for the Non-DoD Schools Program. The DoD Education Activity (DoDEA) oversees the program worldwide through the management of the DoDDS-Europe, DoDDS-Pacific and DDESS Area Offices. The program was established to provide educational guidance and financial support to eligible DoD sponsors assigned to foreign locations to facilitate opportunities for access to available educational programs comparable to that offered in the DoDEA that will support the transition of students to public schools in the United States.

Q. How do I know if my dependent is eligible for educational funding through the NDSP?

A. Eligibility to attend a non-DoD school at government expense is limited to command-sponsored dependents only. A command-sponsored dependent is a minor residing with the active duty military or full-time DoD civilian sponsor at an OCONUS location where an accompanied-by-dependent tour is authorized; the sponsor is authorized to serve that tour, and the dependents meet the following criteria: (1) The dependent is eligible for travel to or from the member's permanent duty station; (2) The dependent is authorized by the appropriate authority to be at the member's permanent duty station; and (3) As a result of the dependent's residence in the vicinity of the sponsor's permanent duty station, the sponsor is entitled to station allowance at the "with family" rate.

Q. How do I enroll my child in a non-DoD School?

A. Contact your local Non-DoD Schools Program (NDSP) liaison. He/She will provide you with a NDSP Application Package containing: (1) Application for Enrollment (DoDEA form 610), (2) Request for Reimbursement of Transportation Expenses, (3) Verification of Eligibility, and (4) Funds Request Sheet (FRS). Each of these forms need to be filled out COMPLETELY and returned to your local NDSP liaison. He/She will forward your completed application package to the NDSP, Program Manager, who will review the package and approve/disapprove eligibility for enrollment. Once you receive notice that your child/children's eligibility for enrollment has/have been approved, THEN, and only then, can you proceed to enroll your child into the non-DoD school of your choice. DDESS MUST APPROVE ELIGIBILITY FOR ENROLLMENT AND FUNDING BEFORE THE CHILD IS ENROLLED IN THE NON-DOD SCHOOL. Enrolling the child prior to approval may result in denial of funds from the NDSP.

Q. How do I know my child will receive a quality education at a non-DoD School? Also, how can we ensure that our child will be placed in the correct grade upon our returning from overseas?

A. Base schools are certified by the Department of State-Office of Overseas Schools to ensure educational standards and curriculums are equivalent to those in U.S. public schools. Parents are entitled, through freedom of choice ("Selection of School," DSR 272.3), to enroll their child/children in a school other than the base school. The responsibility of gathering information on curriculum and educational standards, then comparing that data to the base school, would then be that of the parents and the local NDSP liaison. For children in high school, special attention should be focused on graduation requirements for seniors who will be returning to the United States for their senior year to ensure all graduation requirements are being met. It should be noted that reimbursement for tuition and allowable expenses is limited to that of the base school.

Q. How do I get approval and funding to use home-based educational programs for my child?

A. NDSP liaisons can provide you with a NDSP application package and a list of allowable and nonallowable expenses for home-based education. Once you have completed the application package it should be returned to your NDSP liaison, who will forward it to the NDSP Program Manager for processing. Once approved, the sponsor can begin purchasing materials for use in the home-based educational program. Standard allowance rates for those choosing to home-school their children are K–8, up to $5,700, and 9–12, up to $7,700. Receipts and/or proofs of purchase are required for all items being claimed, and should be submitted to your local NDSP liaison along with a Funds Request Sheet. He/she will submit to the NDSP Program Manager for funding. (SR 274.12.b and SR 277.3.a.)

Q. How do we find the correct information on school policies? How do we ensure that this information is given to the MILGP/USDAOs when a change has been made?

A. The local NDSP liaison is responsible for informing sponsors of changes in program policies. The liaison is responsible for maintaining communications with the local non-DoD schools and their changing school policies. Changes to the NDSP policies and regulations are distributed to all NDSP liaisons by the NDSP Program Manager, and are then distributed to the embassy, commands, and sponsors, as appropriate. Additionally, the NDSP-Americas website has the most up-to-date regulations, policies and forms: www.am.dodea.edu/ndsp.

Q. What if the DSSR for a location isn't enough to cover the costs of tuition and other allowable expenses in our location? How can the embassy get that changed so the parents are not paying out of pocket?

A. The Budget/Finance Office at the U.S. Embassy would need to submit form DS-63 to the State Department, Education Allowances Office, facsimile 202-261-8707. Forms requesting adjustments need to be received by 15 June in order for changes to allowances to be made for the following school year. This office works directly with the embassies to make appropriate adjustments to the DSSR education allowance rates. In cases where a change to the DSSR for a location's education allowance is made midyear, the sponsor will benefit from the higher DSSR rate for the entire school year. Allowable expense amounts that were over the previous DSSR allowance and paid out-of-pocket by the sponsor can be resubmitted and paid under the new DSSR rate.

Q. What are "one time fees"? When are they funded and for how much? How many times they can be claimed?

A. One time fees are nonrefundable fees that the foreign school charges only once per student or per family when initially enrolling in their school and are not charged upon reenrolling in subsequent school years. These fees include, but are not limited to, registration fees, matriculation fees, construction fees, admission fees, infrastructure funds fees, building fees, and so forth.

The NDSP agrees to pay nonrefundable, one time fees equal to the total amount of one time fees charged at the base school. These fees must be listed on the publicized school tuition fee schedule, and they must be fees that are applicable to the local families when they enroll their children. Claims for reimbursement of one time fees do not decrease your amount allowable for tuition and other allowable expenses under the DSSR rate—reimbursement for one time fees are funded in addition to the DSSR education allowance.

"One Time Fees" are just that . . . only paid ONCE during an assignment except in certain cases when:

- A school attended does not offer the next grade (e.g., middle to high school);
- The school attended cannot offer the appropriate programs;
- The school attended is not the base school and charges less than the base school costs, thus, up to the difference between the two costs could be paid should the sponsor elect to change their child's school.

Q. Does the NDSP fund testing and evaluation of services for non-severe learning education needs?

A. State Department Regulation 276.8, "Special Needs Child," states that NDSP will pay for diagnostics testing and for items specifically mandated by a child's Individualized Education Plan (IEP). It should be noted that the DSSR for special needs children is not regulated by country or location. NDSP will reimburse up to $26,800 for special needs education per student, per school year. In addition to the DSSR allowance, funding for tutoring and summer school is reimbursed if deemed mandatory by the child's IEP.

If testing or assessment facilities are not available locally, arrangements can be made through the NDSP for stateside assessment at either a Domestic Dependent Elementary and Secondary School (DDESS) site or through coordination with another medical facility (e.g., Walter Reed). The NDSP is authorized to fund the travel and certain other expenses related to the assessment. Logistical and assessment arrangements are handled directly with the NDSP Program Manager and NDSP Education Support Specialist.

Q. Is there an update on travel authorization for students in the United States to visit home in Latin America?

A. NOTE: This is a trick question! If the students are attending schools in the United States they are not attending a non-DoD school. Therefore, the responsibility for that child to be reimbursed for travel to Latin America from the United States would fall to the military command, not the NDSP. (State Regulation 276.3.)

Q. What financial assistance is available to cover unexpected expenses such as SAT fees ($15 fee to take the test overseas)?

A. SAT and similar testing fees (ACT) are not reimbursable through the NDSP (SR 277, "Allowable Expenses"). PSAT testing fees are reimbursable for 10–11 grade students only. Courses designed for preparation of the PSAT, SAT or ACT are not authorized for reimbursement. The only exception to the regulation would be Advanced Placement (AP) or International Baccalaureate (IB) course-related exams or tests.

Q. How does one enroll a child with special needs in the Non-DoD Schools Program?

A. If you are new to post and this is your first time enrolling your child in the NDSP, you will need to contact your NDSP liaison immediately to facilitate a smooth transition and continuity of services for your dependent. In addition to the NDSP application package, we ask that the sponsor submit any previous documentation to support the identification and services needed to support your child's special needs. This may include copies of previous assessments, Individual Education Plan (IEP) from previous schools, Exceptional Family Member Program (EFMP) reports/assessments or letters or standardized test results from previous schools.

The DSSR Educational Allowance for special needs children is up to $26,800 per school year, per student. In addition to the DSSR, up to $3,000 per school year, per student is allowed for tutoring and summer school—as directly mandated by the IEP. For returning students on an IEP, progress reports may be requested to monitor effectiveness of services. Your NDSP liaison has application/eligibility forms.

Q. Will preschool ever be funded under the NDSP? Some parents are concerned that their child is at a disadvantage as pre-kindergarten is extremely expensive overseas.

A. At this time, preschool is not funded through the NDSP. This decision is based on the fact that in the United States preschool is not mandatory for entry into kindergarten, nor is it provided by U.S. public schools free of charge.

Q. What additional funding support is available for students whose education is funded by SAO or T-20 funds?

A. Students whose tuition and annual fees are funded with SAO or T-20 funding are still eligible for NDSP funding for special education services and/or supplemental instruction needs. Enrollment in the NDSP and supporting documentation of needs is required before funding can be authorized. NDSP liaisons should enroll and track all students receiving educational support in accordance with the NDSP regulations so that supplemental instruction support and special needs support is extended to all eligible sponsors and their dependents.

Q. Why and where in the regulation does it say that PTA charges should be paid by the parents?

A. DoDEA Regulation 1035.1, Enclosure 4, E4.8 Miscellaneous. The reason it is an unauthorized cost for reimbursement is that PTA/PTO dues are a fee that parents pay out of pocket when attending a tax-supported public school in the United States.

Q. The local non-DoD school is requiring uniforms for certain functions this year. Are we authorized reimbursement for these? Its one shirt and one jacket for each child.

A. Uniforms of any kind are an unauthorized expense for reimbursement IAW DoDEA Regulation 1035.1, Enclosure 4, E4.15.

Q. We have an individual whose child has been back in the states living with his mom. A decision was made to have the child move to post to live with dad . . . unexpectedly. The individual is having his sending command amend his order to show command sponsorship. The question is: since he hasn't received those new orders yet and school is starting, can he pay out of pocket now and then get reimbursed for the costs after he receives the orders? Or would he not be eligible until he receives the amended orders?

A. In situations where command-sponsorship of a dependent has been formally requested through the chain of command, the NDSP Program Manager will work with the sending command to verify status of request. Each situation will be reviewed on a case-by-case basis, and every effort will be made to support the educational continuity of the DoD dependent where possible.

Q. For a student receiving a home-based education, are proctoring fees reimbursable? What about fees for extending testing dates due to PCSing?

A. When proof that a proctored test must be administered as part of the home-based educational programs curriculum, proctoring fees will be reimbursed by the NDSP. Additionally, when required testing needs to be rescheduled because of transition issues, the NDSP is authorized to reimburse, within reasonable limits.

Q. I would like to know the NDSP funding policy regarding a student enrolled in a non-DoD school (senior year) whose sponsor has to leave early. Will NDSP pay the entire school year tuition and related fees?

A. Yes. For continuity of education for the dependent, NDSP regulation authorized continued payment of expenses through the completion of the current school year for a dependent whose sponsor transfers during the school year.

Q. Will NDSP approve and fund fees for a religious school?

A. Yes. The parent has the freedom to choose any school they feel best meets the educational needs of their child. However, the reimbursement of educational expenses is limited to the DSSR educational allowance rate. The DSSR rate is typically calculated using the fees charged by the base school. Part of the criteria for a base school is that it does not mandate denominational religious instruction, so it is possible the DSSR rate may not cover all fees incurred. Parents would be responsible for any amounts that exceed the DSSR rate.

5

Medical Care

HEALTH BENEFITS

Understanding TRICARE

Through TRICARE Prime, or TRICARE Prime Remote, two of the health plan options offered through the Department of Defense, most of your basic health-care needs will be met at limited or no charge when enrolled. When needs arise outside of this basic core of care, it is important to be familiar with your options.

For example, if you need care beyond the scope of your primary care manager (PCM), your PCM will evaluate your medical history, current condition, and treatment before referring you to a specialist. This protects the system's limited resources in those cases in which the PCM treatment can meet your medical needs. Once true need is established, you may be referred to a specialist.

If geographically possible, the specialist care will be provided at a military treatment facility (MTF), pending authorization from TRICARE. If you live beyond the reach of an MTF, your provider may refer you automatically. Seeking prior TRICARE approval may be required, depending on the TRICARE option used and your status as a member. When dealing with any health-care system, you may encounter unfamiliar terms and acronyms. Consult the TRICARE glossary to find helpful definitions common to health-care services and organizations.

Authorizations for Care

TRICARE issues an authorization when a TRICARE Prime beneficiary needs specialized medical services only if services are not available at the military treatment facility (MTF) or at the PCM's office. All referrals must be made to network providers. The referral will clearly specify the services authorized, the number of visits, and the time frame in which the visits must be completed.

If you are referred to a specialty provider, you must pay close attention to what is specified on the referral. You may be liable for payment of services you receive beyond what is specified on the referral. For example, if the referral is only for diagnostic testing, that does not authorize you to receive any other care—only the diagnostic test.

Authorizations will be for a certain number of visits and only within a specified duration of time. It is important to keep a calendar of when ongoing visits or authorizations will expire. You will receive statements by mail that provide this information from TRICARE. You are responsible for notifying your PCM of any needed renewals of authorizations or any new prescriptions to continue ongoing specialty care or therapy. Many times medical providers will not notify a patient if their authorization on record has expired, and by pro-actively managing these expirations, you can reduce wait times for having to reschedule with providers and avoid denials of service.

Using the Point-of-Service Option

The TRICARE Prime point-of-service option allows TRICARE Prime enrollees to receive nonemergency, TRICARE-covered services, to include mental health service from any TRICARE-authorized provider without a referral from their primary care manager. Using the TRICARE Prime point-of-service option is more costly to the enrollee.

TRICARE Standard beneficiaries are permitted to seek specialty care from a TRICARE-authorized provider without a referral because that plan option already requires the beneficiaries to pay a higher portion for their care.

There are some procedures that TRICARE generally doesn't cover. For instance, TRICARE Standard does not cover a number of counseling services. You can avoid expensive surprises by checking the details of your coverage before making an appointment.

Specialized Treatment Services

You may be referred for certain high-technology or high-cost procedures to a specialized treatment services facility (STSF). These are facilities established and approved by the government at regional, multiregional, and national levels. Such procedures range from bone marrow or liver transplants to rehabilitation. If you are referred for care, local MTF health benefits advisors or TRICARE health-care finders will assist you with the process.

In some cases, there may be limitations to your coverage. To avoid costly surprises, make sure you understand any possible out-of-pocket expenses before seeking care. If you choose to forego treatment at an STSF when it is available, you will be held responsible for a higher portion or all of the cost of the care you choose.

Receiving Emergency Care

In an emergency, it is not necessary to get prior authorization. Simply go to the nearest military or civilian emergency room or call 911.

Within 24 hours of receiving treatment, contact your PCM or, for active duty members, your service point of contact (SPOC) at the military Medical Support Office. They can help with transferring you to a military hospital, if necessary. They can also help make sure that your medical bills are handled properly.

Supplemental Insurance

To help offset possible costs when using the point-of-service option or specialized treatment services facilities, you might want to examine the possibility of a supplemental insurance plan. These plans are offered by private firms and military associations to help patients not eligible for Medicare with remaining costs after TRICARE pays the government's share. These plans are not individually sponsored or endorsed by the Department of Defense, so carefully consider your needs when purchasing a plan.

Appealing a Claim

If a claim is denied, beneficiaries are encouraged to follow up and find out why. Sometimes a simple clerical error originating in the physician's office is to blame, so it pays to follow through and clear up such errors. If the decision is unchanged, but the beneficiary or provider disagrees, they may appeal the decision.

Only health-care providers who participate in TRICARE can file an appeal; providers cannot file if they don't participate in TRICARE or are not network providers.

The process for appeal will be included with the written decision received by the beneficiary. It generally involves contacting the appropriate regional TRICARE contractor (also listed on the notice of the right to appeal) in writing, within 90 days of the date written on the patient's explanation of benefits (EOB). It is suggested that a copy of the EOB and any other related documents be included, and that beneficiaries keep copies of the paperwork for their own records.

Debt collection assistance officers (DCAO) and beneficiary counseling and assistance coordinators (BCAC), also known as health benefits advisors, are located in TRICARE regional offices and military treatment facilities. If you receive a notice from a collection agency or a negative credit report because of a medical or dental bill, call or visit the nearest DCAO. BCACs are available to assist with other general questions.

When facing a health-care choice, some basic understanding of your options and responsibilities can save both time and money in the long term and ensure that you receive the quality of care you deserve.

Doing your Research

It is essential that you be an effective advocate for your child and this means being able to communicate clearly and unemotionally. Of course, you are going to get emotional because it is your child; but when you have to speak on your child's behalf you have to try to put that aside in order to get your message and concerns across without ambiguity. This is dealt with in more detail further on in this book but there are some points worth mentioning here as far as advocacy and your child's medical treatment is concerned.

The most important thing is to be informed. You need to know as much about your child's condition as possible. You can research your child's condition online, get reference books from your local library, speak to support groups and join local chapters that deal with your child's specific health issues.

You have rights—be sure to know them. While the doctors and medical staff will have you and your child's best interests at heart, their course of action may not always be clear to you and, at times, it might be unacceptable. Study federal, state, and military laws as they relate to special needs medical treatment so that you are informed and can discuss issues knowledgably.

It is better to be part of the team coming up with solutions for your child's care than be regarded as a troublemaker.

Ask Questions

Always ask questions—lots of them. Journalists are trained to ask "who, what, where, when and why." Asking these questions should provide a lot of good information.

Never be afraid to ask questions—always in a polite, nonconfrontational way—and make a note of the answers. If you don't understand why a procedure is being carried out, ask why. If you would like to discuss other options, ask what are available. It pays to have done your research when you get into these sorts of discussions so that you know ahead of time what options you have. If the medical staff don't mention these or dismiss them you have every right to be concerned and ask for a second opinion.

WAIVERS

Important: There are two sorts of waivers. The first is a waiver that can set aside some of the strict eligibility requirements governing income guidelines, benefits, and health-care delivery options required under federal Medicaid program regulations and other forms of medical insurance. The second waiver is the one that informs the medical staff about exemptions of treatment for your child that you are asking for on religious, ethical, and other grounds.

Medicaid Waivers

Children who are not financially eligible for Medicaid or who need additional services beyond those traditionally provided by Medicaid may be eligible for a Medicaid waiver in their state. Each state is required to have a program to assist children with extensive medical needs and disabilities. However, state programs vary widely in eligibility requirements, benefits, and program structure.

In general, states may choose one of two methods for creating a program. The first, often called a "Katie Beckett Waiver" or TEFRA waiver, simply extends regular Medicaid services to children with extensive needs by counting only the child's income and not the income of the parents. These programs are typically only for children who are medically fragile and dependent on technology and would otherwise need institutionalization. States must provide benefits to ALL children who qualify under TEFRA guidelines if they offer a TEFRA waiver, meaning there are no waiting lists.

The second and more common method is for a state to apply to the federal government for an HCBS (Home and Community-Based Services) waiver, often called an HCBS Section 1915(c) waiver. Some states may have both HCBS and TEFRA waivers. HCBS waivers provide traditional Medicaid and additional services, such as nursing, home modification, respite, and behavioral therapy. Most states have multiple programs, including one for children who are medically fragile or physically disabled (if they do not have a TEFRA waiver), another for children with developmental disabilities, and additional specialized programs for children with autism, HIV, or brain injuries.

A Home and Community Based Services Waiver can provide extra services that make living at home possible. This can include personal care, nursing, respite, adult daycare, supported employment, home modifications, assistive technology, and transportation. While waivers can differ substantially between states in eligibility and services, an important advantage is that they can expand services to cover individuals that may be over income for traditional Medicaid. However, because states have the discretion to choose the number of consumers to support in a waiver program, there are often long waiting lists for services.

Personal Waivers

It is important that everyone involved with your child's care—both medical and educational—be aware of your wishes and concerns. For instance, you may have very good reasons for not wanting certain vaccines administered or you may have religious beliefs that you want respected. The medical team will not know these unless you make it known to them.

Vaccines

All states have some requirement that youngsters be immunized against such childhood diseases as measles, mumps, chickenpox, diphtheria, and whooping cough. Twenty-eight states, including Florida, Massachusetts, and New York, allow parents to opt out for medical or religious reasons only. Twenty other states, among them California, Pennsylvania, Texas, and Ohio, also allow parents to cite personal or philosophical reasons. Mississippi and West Virginia allow exemptions for medical reasons only. If you have legitimate reasons for seeking an exemption discuss it with your medical team.

Certain vaccines can be dangerous or inappropriate for children with certain pre-existing medical conditions. For example, the pertussis vaccine is generally regarded as not recommended for children with seizures or a history of seizures. Be sure to consult with your pediatrician, your developmental pediatrician, and other specialists to be sure that if vaccines are expected, that all providers are aware of your child's conditions in order to avoid unnecessary risk to the child. For teenagers, Gardisil, which is a vaccine for human papilloma virus (HPV) does not protect against all strains of HPV, and has the potential for serious side effects. In other words having the vaccine does not guarantee a person cannot contract the virus in this instance. Make sure you are informed about the possible side effects and alleged benefit of any vaccine before allowing your child to receive it, and make informed decisions with your medical providers.

Children who are considered medically fragile may also be candidates for Respiratory Syncytial Virus (RSV) shots, which require special justification from the recommending pediatrician.

Religious Waivers

As above, ensure that people are aware of your religious beliefs and convictions and that these are taken into account by the medical staff and other personnel when treating your child. In some states, you must visit your local county's health department to obtain a form that must be completed and filed in order to protect your particular beliefs and to prevent issues with admission into school districts that otherwise require a full vaccine record that records all inoculations by date for age-appropriate levels.

CASE MANAGEMENT

When Do You Get a Case Manager?

A case manager is usually assigned to assure the provision of coordinated comprehensive services for special needs children and their families. The ultimate goal of the case management unit is to help these families identify and access quality health care so that children have the opportunity to function at their optimum level.

The case manager is a professionally prepared individual and a central figure in the case management system. The case manager serves as a resource for the family regarding the range of service options and entitlements available and to continually assess and evaluate the health-care system to identify gaps that remain to be addressed. The case manager is the mediator between the family and the service delivery system and performs individual service planning, service coordination, and monitoring. All of these functions are carried out with family members.

What Does or Can a Case Manager Do?

The professional case manager works with both children and their parents. These professionals assist families through the maze of the health service system and other related systems and are responsible for providing the following specific services:

- Counseling of the child and parent including: (1) a description of the Special Child Health Service–Case Management Services, (2) identifying the child's problem(s) with the parents, and (3) validating the parents' knowledge and understanding of the child's problem(s).
- Assessing the need for services and developing with the families an Individual Service Plan. This Individual Service Plan is written describ-

ing the child's developmental, educational, medical, rehabilitative, and social needs.

- Assisting families to reach their goals identified in the Individual Service Plan by taking an active part in identifying and accessing the needed service.
- Being available to the families as a resource in a crisis, responding actively to complaints about services, and providing objective information about alternatives for securing direct services.
- Promoting and facilitating communication among multiple providers servicing families including the primary health-care provider.
- Monitoring the services received by families by reviewing the child's progress toward the attainment of goals identified in the Individual Service Plan.

6

Insurance

There is no shortage of options when it comes to health insurance, but most people in the military opt for TRICARE, as it offers many benefits to servicemen and women and their families.

DEPARTMENT OF DEFENSE HEALTH CARE SYSTEM

TRICARE is the Department of Defense's health-care system for members of the military and their families in the United States and all over the world. TRICARE is an organization that includes military health-care resources as well as civilian health-care providers who have been authorized by TRICARE to receive reimbursement. The following are authorized civilian providers: Network providers who have discount agreements with TRICARE. Participating providers who are not part of the TRICARE network but who have agreed to accept TRICARE allowable charges as payment in full. Nonparticipating providers who do not accept TRICARE allowable charges as payment in full. These providers may be paid up to 15 percent more than the allowable charges and may require beneficiaries to file their own claims and wait for reimbursement.

TRICARE is organized into four geographic regions: North, South, West, and Overseas. The three regions located within the United States offer the same options for health-care plans and coverage. If you are a TRICARE beneficiary living overseas, you have fewer options. Visit the TRICARE website, www.tricare.mil, to find helpful links to TRICARE regional websites.

TRICARE Standard is the TRICARE option that provides the most flexibility to TRICARE-eligible beneficiaries. It is the fee-for-service option that gives beneficiaries the opportunities to see any TRICARE-authorized provider. TRICARE Standard is not available to active duty service members. Standard shares most of the costs of medically necessary care from civilian providers when military treatment facility (MTF) care is unavailable.

All active duty service members are eligible for TRICARE Prime. However they must fill out an enrollment form and submit it to the regional contractor. In addition, service members receive most of their care from military medical personnel. For active duty families, there is no enrollment fee for TRICARE Prime; however, they must complete an enrollment form to select Prime as their coverage plan.

With TRICARE Prime, most health care will come from a military treatment facility (MTF), along with the TRICARE contracted Civilian Medical Providers called Preferred Provider Network (PPN).

With TRICARE Extra, you don't have to enroll or pay an annual fee. You do have to satisfy an annual deductible for outpatient care, just as you do under TRICARE Standard. The deductible and cost-sharing work the same way for TRICARE Extra. In the TRICARE Extra program, when you receive care from a TRICARE Extra network provider, you get a discount on cost-sharing, and you don't have to file your own claims. You don't enroll and may use TRICARE Extra on a case-by-case basis just by using the network providers. TRICARE Extra is not available overseas or to active duty service members.

TRICARE OPTIONS FOR ACTIVE DUTY FAMILY MEMBERS

To meet the diverse needs of active duty families, TRICARE offers several health-care plans.

TRICARE Prime

Prime is TRICARE's managed-care option, similar to a civilian health maintenance organization. Active duty service members are required to be enrolled in TRICARE Prime and may choose to enroll their families. This is the only TRICARE option that requires enrollment and the service member must enroll each family member. The beneficiaries receive medical care from a local military treatment facility or from a network approved health-care provider. Active duty family members who are enrolled in Prime enjoy enhanced clinical preventive benefits. As a Prime enrollee, you must follow some well-defined rules and procedures, such as seeking care first from your primary care manager and receiving a referral from him or her as well as authorization from your regional contractor when seeking specialty care. Failure to follow these steps may result in costly Point of Service (POS) charges.

The TRICARE Prime Point-of-Service option (POS) allows TRICARE Prime enrollees to receive nonemergency TRICARE-covered services from any TRI-CARE-authorized provider without a referral from their primary care manager or authorization from a health-care finder. Using the TRICARE PRIME point-of-service option is more costly to the enrollee and POS charges incurred after the catastrophic cap has been met are the beneficiary's responsibility.

TRICARE Prime Remote

If you are a family member living with an active duty service person, and you live either 50 miles or a 1-hour drive from the closest military medical treatment facility, you may enroll in TRICARE Prime Remote for Active Duty Family Members. Enrollment is required, and once enrolled you must select or be assigned a local primary care manager (PCM) where network primary care providers are available. If no network primary care provider is available, you may use any TRICARE authorized provider for primary care. Contact your TRICARE regional managed care support contractor for help locating a provider.

TRICARE Standard

Standard is a fee-for-service option that gives eligible family members the option to see any TRICARE-certified/authorized provider (e.g., doctor, nurse-practitioner, lab, clinic, etc.).

TRICARE Standard can be used simultaneously with Extra (discussed in following section). If you see a non-network provider you will incur greater out-of-pocket costs and have to file your own claims. However, Standard affords you the greatest choice of providers and may be the only option to family members in some locations. It is not an option for active duty service members. To see a cost comparison of TRICARE options see the chart at www.tricare.mil/mybenefit/home/overview/ComparePlans.

TRICARE Extra

TRICARE Extra is a preferred-provider option that allows active duty family members using the TRICARE Standard benefit to receive care from TRI-CARE network providers with lower out-of-pocket costs.

With TRICARE Extra there are no claims to file, but the choice of providers is limited to those in the network. TRICARE Extra is not available to active duty members, nor is it available overseas.

Pharmacy Benefit

The TRICARE pharmacy benefit offers multiple ways to have a prescription filled. The most cost-effective way to receive prescription drugs is through the nearest uniformed services military medical treatment facility (MTF). If unable to visit a uniformed services MTF pharmacy, you have three other options: TRICARE mail order pharmacy (TMOP), TRICARE retail network pharmacies, and non-network pharmacies. For more information on how to save costs and make the most of this benefit visit www.tricare.mil/mybenefit/home/Prescriptions/PharmacyProgram.

TRICARE'S BENEFITS FOR FAMILIES WITH SPECIAL NEEDS

To help families in the military who face the extra challenges that come with caring for a special needs family member, TRICARE offers additional programs to those who are eligible.

Extended Care Health Option (ECHO)

In 2005, TRICARE introduced the Extended Care Health Option (ECHO) to replace the Program For Persons With Disabilities (PFPWD). TRICARE ECHO offers most of the benefits that PFPWD did, with the addition of home respite care and an increase in the allowable cost share from the government from $1,000 to $2,500. The purpose of the ECHO program is to provide financial assistance and additional benefits for services, equipment, or supplies beyond those available through TRICARE Prime, Extra, or Standard.

Who Qualifies?

Active duty family members who have one of the following conditions may qualify for ECHO benefits:

Moderate or severe mental retardation.
A serious physical disability.
An extraordinary physical or psychological condition that leaves the beneficiary homebound.

Multiple disabilities involving two or more body systems.

How Do I Register?

To participate in TRICARE ECHO the beneficiary must first do the following:

Enroll in the Exceptional Family Member Program (EFMP) of the sponsor's Military Service.
Once enrolled in EFMP, register with the regional TRICARE office.

You can enroll in the Exceptional Family Member Program at your nearest Family Support Center. To find this go to www.militaryinstallations.dod.mil. Here you will be able to find your nearest Family Support Center and a point of contact for the EFMP.

To enroll in EFMP you must complete Department of Defense (DoD) form 2792, which is a medical summary, and if your child is school age you must also complete DoD form 2792-1, which is a summary of special education or early intervention services. Submit these completed forms to your EFMP coordinator for processing. Once form 2792 is completed and approved by the EFMP coordinator, you must then show proof of enrollment to the Managed Care Support Contractor (MCSC). In most cases, a copy of the approved 2792 form is considered proof. The MCSC is the one who will approve ECHO coverage and update the DEERS system to indicate that your child is eligible for ECHO. You can expect this process to take four to six weeks.

In the meantime, contact the Regional TRICARE contractor with proof of enrollment in EFMP. The proof of enrollment can be a copy of your application form for EFMP.

Eligible family members may be granted provisional ECHO status for a period of no more than 90 days while they wait for their application to be completed.

What Benefits Are Available?

The following are ECHO benefits:

Medical and rehabilitative services, prostheses, orthopedic braces, and appliances.
Durable equipment and maintenance.
Training for families to use assistive technology devices.
Training for families to provide home administered medical interventions.
Special education.

Institutional care when residential care is required.

Transportation under certain conditions.

Assistive communication services (e.g., interpreters, readers for the blind).

16 hours of respite care services per month if the beneficiary is receiving another ECHO benefit.

ECHO Home Health Care (see next section).

Respite Care

Some families are interested in respite care but are concerned about the individuals who will care for their child in their absence. Respite care providers are all hired through Medicare certified home health agencies. This means that there have been background checks and screening done to help assure the quality of the caregivers. Meet your caregiver before they care for your child to determine your comfort level with the individual. If the caregiver does not seem to be a good fit for your family, ask for another applicant from the agency.

Certified home health agencies often face shortages of qualified personnel. There may be a significant wait time between filing a request for the provision of a caregiver and receiving someone who is both qualified and acceptable to work with the EFM in the home.

ECHO Cost Shares

Sponsors will pay part of the monthly authorized ECHO expenses for their family members based on their pay grade (table 6.1).

After the monthly cost share is paid, TRICARE will pay up to $2,500 per month for authorized ECHO benefits, except for the ECHO Home (EHHC) benefit. If costs exceed $2,500 per month, the sponsor is responsible for the additional costs. If more than one family member with the same sponsor qualifies for ECHO, TRICARE will pay up to $2,500 for each eligible beneficiary.

ECHO Home Healthcare (EHHC)

EHHC provides homebound family members with intensive home services and supplies if they generally require more than 28 hours per week of home health services or respite care.

Beneficiaries are considered homebound if their condition generally prevents them from being able to go out because of the considerable and taxing effort of leaving the home.

Table 6.1

ECHO Cost-Shares	
Sponsor Pay Grade	Monthly Cost-Share
E-1 through E-5	$25.00
E-6	$30.00
E-7 and O-1	$35.00
E-8 and O-2	$40.00
E-9, WO/WO-1, CWO-2, and O-3	$45.00
CWO-3, CWO-4, and O-4	$50.00
CWO-5, O-5	$65.00
O-6	$75.00
O-7	$100.00
O-8	$150.00
O-9	$200.00
O-10	$250.00

Any absence of the beneficiary due to treatments or adult daycare programs will not disqualify beneficiaries from being considered homebound and eligible for EHHC. This can be of use to beneficiaries who stay home to avoid living in institutional facilities, acute care facilities, or skilled nursing homes.

Your child may qualify for the following benefits:

Nursing care from a registered nurse or by a licensed or vocational nurse who is under the direct supervision of a registered nurse.

Services provided by a home health aid under the direct supervision of a registered nurse.

Physical therapy, occupational therapy, speech and language services, or medical or social services under the direction of a physician.

Teaching and training activities.

Medical supplies.

How Do I Qualify for EHHC?

To qualify for EHHC the family member must meet all of the following requirements:

Be registered in ECHO.

Physically reside in the United States, the District of Columbia, Puerto
Rico, the Virgin Islands, or Guam.

Be homebound.

Be case managed, to include required services as specified in a physician
certified plan of care, and receive periodic assessments of needs.

Receive home services from a TRICARE authorized home agency.

Require medically necessary skilled services beyond the level of coverage
provided by the TRICARE Home Prospective Payment System benefit.

Require more than two medical interventions during the 8-hour period that
the primary caregiver(s) would normally be sleeping.

EHHC Respite Benefit

Respite care is a break from duty for parents of specially challenged children.
This benefit is offered to help primary caregivers as well as their children. It
provides rest for parents as well as skilled supervision for children. The goal
is to promote well-being for the whole family. This benefit is geared to help
families with homebound children who have medical conditions that require
frequent interventions by their primary caregivers. These beneficiaries may
receive 8 hours of respite care 5 days a week. A Medicare certified home
health agency will provide information on caregivers, whom you can meet
before they care for your child. It is intended for family members whose medical conditions require frequent interventions, so that the primary caregiver
has time to sleep. This is separate from the 16 hours of respite care offered
by ECHO and cannot be used with the ECHO respite care program. Respite
benefits cannot be used for sibling care, employment, deployment, or pursu-
ing education, and they are not accumulative.

Home Health Care

Home health care may be authorized for an active duty family instead of
EHHC if the need is intermittent or part-time. Services include skilled nursing and home health aid care.

Skilled Nursing Facility Care

TRICARE will provide coverage for care delivered in a skilled nursing facility (SNF) when nursing and rehabilitation services are determined to be medically necessary. They are provided by licensed nurses, physical therapists, occupational therapists, and so forth, and they are performed under the general
supervision of a Medicare/TRICARE-authorized physician. For TRICARE to

cover your child's admission to a skilled nursing facility, the child must have had a medical condition that required hospitalization for at least 3 consecutive days. Admission to the skilled nursing facility is covered as long as your child is admitted within 30 days of discharge from the hospital. Your doctor's plan of care must demonstrate your child's need for medically necessary, skilled services for TRICARE to pay for the care.

Hospice Care

Hospice care is designed to comfort terminally ill patients and their families once the patient is not expected to live longer than 6 months. The goal of hospice care is to provide dignity and comfort to the dying, and 80 percent of hospice care takes place at home or in nursing homes. TRICARE will cover most of the costs of hospice care, and there are no limits on custodial care or personal comfort items under hospice rules. Beneficiaries must elect hospice in lieu of basic benefits.

Mental Health Care

Unless the beneficiary has a serious mental illness that qualifies for care under ECHO, mental health-care benefits can be confusing. Mental health-care covered under the TRICARE program has the following restrictions.

The provider must establish the medical necessity, and the TRICARE contractor must pre-authorize the following mental health-care services:

Inpatient care, up to authorized annual limit
Care at residential treatment facilities
Extensions to TRICARE annual limits on inpatient care
Outpatient mental care exceeding 2 outpatient visits per week or 8 outpatient visits per year

The following are annual limits for inpatient care:

30 days for patients over age 19
45 days for patients under age 19
150 days for inpatient care in residential treatment centers (available only to those under age 21)
7 days' detox and 21 days' rehabilitation for substance abuse

The disorders that qualify for TRICARE mental health-care benefits include conditions such as depression, anxiety, obsessive-compulsive disorder, bi-polar disorder, schizophrenia, attention deficit disorders, and autism.

TRICARE mental health benefits do not cover treatment for weight loss, sexual dysfunction, certain personality disorders, or special learning disabilities.

Case Management

Case management is offered as a system for organizing and integrating the many services that are often required for the management of complex physical or emotional illnesses. It is designed to improve the quality of care, control costs, and support patients through catastrophic medical situations by providing a bridge between acute-care and long-term-care services. TRICARE offers case management to beneficiaries who are receiving care for chronic or high risk health issues. Beneficiaries with catastrophic or terminal illnesses may also qualify for case management. If you are interested in case management, ask your primary care provider for information.

Help and Information

You can access the TRICARE program twenty-four hours a day, seven days a week by visiting the TRICARE website, (www.tricare.mil). From the site you can get regional contractor contact information, including toll-free numbers and links to region-specific Web pages. You can find important TRICARE information and get your questions answered regarding eligibility, TRICARE Prime enrollment, benefits and co-payments, services that require a referral or prior authorization, claims payment, and any other type of TRICARE question.

Should you need help with TRICARE issues, have all information about your case at hand when you talk to a customer service representative or your case manager. This includes referrals and authorizations, TRICARE Explanation of Benefits (EOBs), medical/dental bills from providers, letters regarding denials, and debt collection notices. The information you provide will help your case manager move quickly to understand and resolve your problem. The representatives/case managers will work with you and provide other agency points of contact to help you with your case.

TRICARE Service Center (TSC) Directory

TSCs are located throughout the regions and are staffed with customer service representatives to provide help on a walk-in basis. There is a TSC locator available through the TRICARE website.

Beneficiary Counseling and Assistance Coordinators (BCACs)/Health Benefits Advisors (HBAs)

Regional offices and most military treatment facilities are staffed with beneficiary counselors/benefit advisors whose job is to advocate for you and advise you about the TRICARE system. These counselors can provide information assistance on benefit options, enrollment questions, status of claims information, as well as help with referrals and appointments. The benefits counselor can aid communication between beneficiaries and the military treatment facility and help find answers to questions that can't be found through the usual channels, as well as help with the appeals process. There is a BCAC Directory at www.tricare.mil.bcacdcao.

Debt Collection Assistance Office Program

TRICARE provides Debt Collection and Assistance Officers (DCAO) whose role it is to advocate for beneficiaries who need help dealing with the confusion of multiple medical or dental bills. If you have received a notice from a collection agency concerning a medical bill or have a dispute about a medical bill, do not hesitate to contact the closest DCAO. They will help research your claim and provide you with a written explanation of how to resolve your collection problem.

Should you need the assistance of a DCAO, you should bring any documentation you have concerning the collection action or billing dispute. This includes debt collection letters, TRICARE Explanation of Benefits (EOBs), and medical/dental bills from providers. The more information you can provide, the easier it will be to determine the cause of the problem.

The DCAO will research your claim with the appropriate claims processor or other agency points of contact and provide you with a written explanation of how to resolve your collection problem. The collection agency will be notified by the DCAO that action is being taken to resolve the issue.

The DCAO cannot provide you with legal advice or fix your credit rating, but it can help you through the debt collection process by providing you with documentation for your use with the collection or credit reporting agency in explaining the circumstances relating to the debt. You may locate the nearest DCAO by contacting your TRICARE contractor or online at www.tricare.mil.bcacdcao.

Catastrophic Cap

The TRICARE catastrophic cap limits the amount of out-of-pocket expenses a family will have to pay for TRICARE–covered medical services. The cap applies to all allowable charges for covered services to include annual deductibles, Prime enrollment fees, pharmacy co-pays, and other TRICARE allowable cost shares. Not included are out-of-pocket expenses paid under TRICARE Prime Point of Service option (POS). Also, any POS charges incurred after the catastrophic cap has been met are the beneficiaries' responsibility.

For Prime enrollees the catastrophic cap for active duty members and their families is $1,000. For families using Standard and Extra the catastrophic cap is $1,000 for family members of active duty service members and $3,000 for other beneficiaries.

IDEA and TRICARE

The Individuals with Disabilities Education Act (IDEA) is legislation that ensures all children with disabilities are provided with a free and appropriate public education (FAPE). This includes services necessary to meet the educational goals described in their Individual Education Program (IEP). Infants and toddlers who are, or may become, delayed due to impairment may receive Early Intervention Services (EIS) or Educational Developmental and Intervention Services (EDIS) if they are in a DoD school system. The services these children receive are often medical, diagnostic, or therapeutic in nature and are provided by health-care providers. These services must be identified either in an Individual Family Service Plan (ISFP) or an Individual Education Program (IEP). IDEA policy intends for these services to be provided at little or no cost to families.

The most recent legislation stipulates that TRICARE will pay its share of early intervention services that are medically or psychologically necessary and would otherwise be a TRICARE benefit. Cost-sharing decisions are made on a case-by-case basis. Services identified in an IEP for special education students between the ages of 3 and 21 are paid for by state educational agencies, and TRICARE will be involved only when it can be shown that the necessary services are not available or adequate to meet the child's needs.

TRIWEST

TriWest Healthcare Alliance is a privately held company based in Phoenix and contracted by the Department of Defense (DoD) to administer the TRICARE program in the 21-state West Region.

TRICARE is available to our nation's active duty, guard and reserve, and retired uniformed service members and their eligible family members and survivors. TriWest received its first DoD TRICARE contract in 1996, then received a 4-year contract extension in 2002. TriWest was awarded a 5-year contract to administer TRICARE in the West Region in 2003, and now provides access to health care for approximately 2.7 million beneficiaries.

The TRICARE West Region covers 2,288,309 square miles and includes the states listed in table 6.2. The terms "TriWest" and "TRICARE" are often used interchangeably, but each is distinctly different. It's easy to see why people may be confused—the names of both start with the same three letters, and both have similar logos.

TRICARE is not an insurance plan, but rather a health-care entitlement earned by our nation's military members for their service to this country. Likewise, TriWest is not an insurance company. TriWest is a contractor to the DoD that administers the TRICARE program in the 21-state West Region.

Table 6.2

1	Alaska
2	Arizona
3	California
4	Colorado
5	Hawaii
6	Idaho
7	Iowa[1]
8	Kansas
9	Minnesota
10	Missouri[2]
11	Montana
12	Nebraska
13	Nevada
14	New Mexico
15	North Dakota
16	Oregon
17	South Dakota
18	Texas[3]
19	Utah
20	Washington
21	Wyoming

1 Excluding the Rock Island Arsenal area.
2 Excluding certain ZIP codes in the St. Louis area.
3 Serving only a portion of western Texas including the El Paso and Fort Bliss area

For more information go to www.triwest.com.

PRIVATE HEALTH-CARE COVERAGE

Other types of health-care coverage available privately include:

Disability Income Insurance

Disability income (DI) insurance pays benefits to individuals who lose their ability to work due to injury or illness. DI insurance replaces income lost while the policyholder is unable to work during a period of disability (in contrast to medical expense insurance, which pays for the cost of medical care). For most working-age adults, the risk of disability is greater than the risk of premature death, and the resulting reduction in lifetime earnings can be significant. Private disability insurance is sold on both a group and an individual basis. Policies may be designed to cover long-term disabilities (LTD coverage) or short-term disabilities (STD coverage). Business owners can also purchase disability overhead insurance to cover the overhead expenses of their business while they are unable to work.

A basic level of disability income protection is provided through the Social Security Disability Insurance (SSDI) program for qualified workers who are totally and permanently disabled (the worker is incapable of engaging in any "substantial gainful work," and the disability is expected to last at least 12 months or result in death).

Long-term Care Insurance

Long-term care (LTC) insurance reimburses the policyholder for the cost of long-term or custodial care services designed to minimize or compensate for the loss of functioning due to age, disability, or chronic illness. LTC has many surface similarities to long-term disability insurance. There are at least two fundamental differences, however. LTC policies cover the cost of certain types of chronic care, while long-term-disability policies replace income lost while the policyholder is unable to work. For LTC, the event triggering benefits is the need for chronic care, while the triggering event for disability insurance is the inability to work.

Private LTC insurance is growing in popularity in the United States. Premiums have remained relatively stable in recent years. However, the coverage is quite expensive, especially when consumers wait until retirement age to purchase it. The average age of new purchasers was 61 in 2005, and has been dropping.

Supplemental Coverage

Private insurers offer a variety of supplemental coverages in both the group and individual markets. These are not designed to provide the primary source of medical or disability protection for an individual, but can assist with unexpected expenses and provide additional peace of mind for those insured. Supplemental coverages include Medicare supplement insurance, hospital indemnity insurance, dental insurance, vision insurance, accidental death and dismemberment insurance, and specified disease insurance.

Supplemental coverages are intended to:

- Supplement a primary medical expense plan by paying for expenses that are excluded or subject to the primary plan's cost-sharing requirements (e.g., co-payments, deductibles, etc.);
- Cover related expenses such as dental or vision care;
- Assist with additional expenses that may be associated with a serious illness or injury.

Medicare Supplement Coverage (Medigap)

Medicare Supplement policies are designed to cover expenses not covered (or only partially covered) by the "original Medicare" (Parts A and B) fee-for-service benefits. They are only available to individuals enrolled in Medicare Parts A and B. Medigap plans may be purchased on a guaranteed issue basis (no health questions asked) during a 6-month open enrollment period when an individual first becomes eligible for Medicare. The benefits offered by Medigap plans are standardized.

Hospital Indemnity Insurance

Hospital indemnity insurance provides a fixed daily, weekly, or monthly benefit while the insured is confined in a hospital. The payment is not dependent on actual hospital charges, and is most commonly expressed as a flat dollar amount. Hospital indemnity benefits are paid in addition to any other benefits that may be available, and are typically used to pay out-of-pocket and non-covered expenses associated with the primary medical plan, and to help with additional expenses (e.g., child care) incurred while in the hospital.

FEDERAL AND STATE PROGRAMS WITH BENEFITS FOR SPECIAL NEEDS FAMILIES

The federal, state, and local governments offer programs designed to aid disabled children and to ensure they receive the medical and educational assistance they need. These benefits may be used by military families to augment TRICARE benefits, and several are listed here.

Supplemental Security Income (SSI)

SSI is a monthly payment to those with low incomes and few resources, and who are disabled, blind, or 65 or older. Children may qualify. If you think you or your child might qualify, visit your nearest Social Security Office or call the Social Security Administration Office at 1-800-772-1213.

Medicaid

Medicaid is a program that pays for some individuals and families with low income and few resources. Military families who are struggling with the cost of care for a disabled family member should apply for Medicaid. Benefits may exceed those offered by TRICARE. To apply, go to www.cms.hhs.gov.

Medicare

Medicare is a basic health insurance program for Americans over the age of 65 and those with disabilities. Qualification for Medicare is based on the Medicare tax paid through work; however, a worker's spouse, minor children, and disabled adult children may also qualify. To learn more, contact www.medicare.gov.

Food Stamps and Women, Infants, and Children (WIC)

Food stamps and WIC are programs designed to provide families with low incomes a nutritious diet. Eligibility is based on income and resources. TRICARE manages a WIC program for Active Duty Family Members (ADFMs) who are overseas. For information about these nutrition programs, contact www.fns.usda.gov.

Extended Health Care Option (ECHO)

The Extended Care Health Option (ECHO) provides financial assistance to eligible beneficiaries who qualify, based on specific mental or physical disabilities, and offers services and supplies not available through the basic TRICARE program. ECHO supplements the benefits of the basic TRICARE program option that eligible family members use.

ECHO is a supplemental program to the basic TRICARE program. ECHO provides financial assistance for an integrated set of services and supplies to eligible active duty family members (including family members of activated National Guard or Reserve members).

There is no enrollment fee for ECHO, however family members must:

- Have an ECHO-qualifying condition.
- Enroll in the Exceptional Family Member Program (EFMP) as provided by the sponsor's branch of service.
- Register in ECHO through ECHO case managers in each TRICARE region.

Other Benefits under ECHO

ECHO's additional components include respite care and ECHO's Home Health Care (EHHC). ECHO also addresses the needs of the caregiver, which, in most cases, involves rest or time away from the "care environment."

Respite Care

Respite care provides relief for caregivers of special needs dependents. ECHO beneficiaries qualify for 16 hours of respite care a month, to be administered in the home by a TRICARE authorized home health agency. During respite hours, the caregiver may leave the home. Note that respite care is authorized only when the beneficiary is receiving some other ECHO benefit during the same month.

ECHO's Home Health Care

ECHO also includes extended home health care and respite care for caregivers of special needs dependents whose condition renders them homebound. EHHC allows for licensed or registered nurses to provide skilled home health care in excess of 28 hours a week. Speak to your regional contractor or TRICARE Area Office to determine the maximum monthly limit (cap) for EHHC home care benefits.

Respite care under EHHC allows for a maximum of 8 hours, 5 days per week of respite care, which may be used as a sleep benefit. Respite care under EHHC cannot be used in conjunction with ECHO's respite care.

Finally, the monthly benefits maximum has increased from $1,000 to $2,500. In addition, the cost-share liability was not adjusted. Monthly cost-shares range from $25 to $250, depending on the sponsor's pay grade (see table 6.1).

Eligibility and Enrollment

Families are required to be enrolled in their Service's Exceptional Family Member Program in order to register for ECHO benefits. If you qualify for special needs benefits, speak to an EFMP representative, who will ensure your proper enrollment in EFMP and provide appropriate ECHO contact information.

In order to qualify for ECHO benefits, dependents of an active duty service member must have a qualifying condition. Contact your regional managed care support contractor to determine program eligibility and details.

For further information regarding ECHO and EHHC, visit www.tricare. mil/echo or call your TRICARE Regional Office (TRO):

North Region: 1-877-874-2273
South Region: 1-800-444-5445
West Region: 1-888-874-9378
Overseas: 1-888-777-8343

Enhanced Access to Autism Services Demonstration

Several treatments, therapies, and interventions, known as Educational Interventions for Autism Spectrum Disorders (EIA), are available and they have been shown to reduce or eliminate specific problem behaviors and teach new skills to individuals with autism.

These EIA services are not covered under basic TRICARE coverage (TRICARE Prime, TRICARE Standard and Extra, etc.), and are only partially covered through the Extended Care Health Option (ECHO). The Enhanced Access to Autism Services Demonstration allows eligible beneficiaries to have access to a greater range of existing evidence-based EIA services through an expanded network of educational intervention providers.

The Enhanced Access to Autism Services Demonstration is only available in the fifty United States and the District of Columbia. Visit the TRICARE Autism Services Demonstration website for additional information.

Scheduled Health Insurance Plans

Scheduled health insurance plans are an expanded form of hospital indemnity plans. In recent years, these plans have been called mini-med plans or association plans. These plans may provide benefits for hospitalization, surgical, and physician services; however, they are not meant to replace a traditional comprehensive health insurance plan. Scheduled health insurance plans are more of a basic policy providing access to day-to-day health care such as going to the doctor or getting a prescription drug; but these benefits will be limited and are not meant to be effective for catastrophic events. Payments are based on the plan's "schedule of benefits" and are usually paid directly to the service provider. These plans cost much less than comprehensive health insurance. Annual benefit maximums for a typical scheduled health insurance plan may range from $1,000 to $25,000.

TRICARE for Life (TFL)

If you are currently entitled or will soon become entitled to Medicare, there is some important information you should know about your TRICARE coverage. When you become entitled to Medicare Part A and have Medicare Part B coverage, you also become entitled to TRICARE For Life (TFL) benefits.

TFL is TRICARE's Medicare wraparound coverage, which means TRICARE pays secondary to Medicare for TRICARE-covered services. If you are entitled to Medicare Part A due to age, disability, or end-stage renal disease, you must also have Medicare Part B coverage to be eligible for TFL. If you are an active duty family member, you are not required to have Medicare Part B coverage to remain eligible for TRICARE.

If you have Medicare Part A only, you may enroll in Medicare Part B during the general enrollment period, which runs from 1 January to 31 March each year. Part B coverage will begin on 1 July of the year you enroll. For more information about enrolling in Medicare Part B: Call 1-800-772-1213 or visit the Social Security Administration (SSA) online at www.ssa.gov.

Updating DEERS Triggers TFL Eligibility

The Defense Enrollment Eligibility Reporting System (DEERS) receives Medicare entitlement information from the Centers for Medicare and Medicaid Services monthly for beneficiaries ages 65 and older and quarterly for beneficiaries younger than 65 years of age. It's important to verify that your information has been updated because your information in DEERS is what triggers your TFL eligibility.

You can verify your DEERS information in several ways: by phone, fax, mail, and Internet.

What TFL Covers

Here's how TRICARE and Medicare work together to provide you with coverage:

- For services covered by both Medicare and TRICARE, Medicare pays first and TRICARE pays second—you pay nothing.
- For services covered by TRICARE but not Medicare, TRICARE will pay its portion, and you are responsible for applicable TRICARE deductibles and cost-shares (the same as what you would pay for TRICARE Standard or Extra).
- For services covered by Medicare but not TRICARE, Medicare will pay its portion, and you are responsible for Medicare deductibles and cost-shares.
- For services not covered by Medicare or TRICARE, you are responsible for the entire bill.

Getting Care

You can seek care from any Medicare participating or nonparticipating provider. A participating provider agrees to "accept assignment," which means he or she agrees to accept the Medicare approved payment as payment in full for Part B services and supplies. TRICARE For Life will pay the co-insurance and deductibles.

A nonparticipating provider is a provider that does not accept assignment. His or her charges are often higher. Nonparticipating providers are subject to the "limiting charge," which means they cannot charge more than 115 percent of the Medicare approved amount.

TRICARE For Life will pay its portion, up to 115 percent of the Medicare approved amount. Most Medicare providers are also TRICARE authorized, but you can check with your regional contractor to see if your provider is TRICARE authorized, or you can visit the TRICARE Standard Provider Resources page at www.tricare.mil/standardprovider/.

If you become eligible for TFL and are currently seeing a provider who accepts TRICARE, you should check to see if they are a Medicare participating or nonparticipating provider—otherwise, you could be responsible for costs of care you receive.

TRICARE: Interpreting Authorizations

TRICARE covers most inpatient and outpatient care that is medically necessary and considered proven. However, there are special rules or limits on certain types of care, while other types of care are not covered at all. Some military treatment facilities (MTFs) may offer services, procedures, or benefits that are not necessarily covered under TRICARE. You should contact your local MTF for more information. To find an MTF near you, visit the MTF Locator on the TRICARE website at www.tricare.osd.mil/mtf.

A prior authorization is a process of reviewing medical, surgical, and behavioral health services to ensure medical or psychological necessity and appropriateness of care prior to services being rendered. Prior authorizations must be obtained prior to services being rendered or within 24 hours of an admission.

Ensuring Your Visits and Dates on Your Authorizations Are Current

TRICARE issues an authorization when a TRICARE Prime beneficiary needs specialized medical services only if services are not available at the military treatment facility (MTF) or at the PCM's office. All referrals must be made to network providers. The referral will clearly specify the services authorized, the number of visits, and the time frame in which the visits must be completed.

Authorizations will be for a certain number of visits and only within a specified duration of time. It is important to keep a calendar of when ongoing visits or authorizations will expire. You will receive statements by mail that provide this information from TRICARE. You are responsible for notifying your PCM of any needed renewals of authorizations or any new prescriptions to continue ongoing specialty care or therapy. Many times medical providers will not notify a patient if their authorization on record has expired, and by pro-actively managing these expirations, you can reduce wait times for having to re-schedule with providers and avoid denials of service.

Payments and Co-pays

Beneficiaries are responsible for cost-shares and deductibles for care that is covered under TRICARE Standard and Extra. Providers who participate in TRICARE will accept the TRICARE allowable charge (TAC) as the full fee for services they render. However, nonparticipating providers may charge up to 15 percent above the TAC for their services, and TRICARE Standard beneficiaries are financially responsible for these additional charges.

Beware of Billing Procedures

A TRICARE Explanation of Benefits (EOB) is a statement sent to you showing what action has been taken on your TRICARE claims. An EOB is sent to you for your information and files. An EOB is not a bill. After reviewing the EOB, you have the right to appeal certain decisions regarding your claims and must do so in writing within 90 days of the date of the EOB notice. You should keep EOBs with your health insurance records for reference.

How to Read Your TRICARE EOB

PGBA, LLC—PGBA processes all TRICARE claims for the region where you live.

Prime Contractor—The name of your prime contractor.

Date of Notice—PGBA prepared your TRICARE explanation of benefits (EOB) on this date.

Sponsor SSN/Sponsor Name—Your claim is processed using the Social Security number (SSN) of the military service member (active duty, retired, or deceased) who is your TRICARE sponsor. For security reasons, only the last four digits of your SSN will appear on the EOB.

Beneficiary Name—The patient who received medical care and for whom this claim was filed.

Mail-to Name and Address—The EOB is mailed directly to the patient (or patient's parent or guardian) at the address given on the claim. (**Note:** Be sure your doctor has updated your records with your current address.)

Benefits Were Payable to—This field will appear only if your doctor accepts assignment. This means the doctor accepts the TRICARE allowable charge as payment in full for the services you received.

Claim Number—Each claim is assigned a unique number. This helps keep track of the claim as it is processed. It also helps find the claim quickly whenever you call or write with questions or concerns.

Service Provided by/Date of Services— This section lists who provided your medical care, the number of services and the procedure codes, as well as the date you received the care.

Services Provided—This section describes the medical services you received and how many services are itemized on your claim. It also lists the specific procedure codes that doctors, hospitals, and labs use to identify the specific medical services you received.

Amount Billed—Your doctor, hospital, or lab charged this fee for the medical services you received.

TRICARE Approved—This is the amount TRICARE approves for the services you received.

See Remarks—If you see a code or a number here, look at the Remarks section (17) for more information about your claim.

Claim Summary—Here you get a detailed explanation of the action taken on your claim. You will find the following totals: amount billed, amount approved by TRICARE, noncovered amount, amount that you have already paid to the provider (if any), amount your primary health insurance paid (if TRICARE is your secondary insurance), benefits TRICARE has paid to the provider, benefits TRICARE has paid to the beneficiary. A check number will appear here only if a check accompanies your EOB.

Beneficiary Liability Summary—You may be responsible for a portion of the fee your doctor has charged. If so, you'll see that amount itemized here. It will include any charges that have been applied to your annual deductible and any cost-share or co-payment you must pay.

Benefit Period Summary—This section shows how much of the individual and family annual deductible and maximum out-of-pocket expense you have met to date. If you are a TRICARE Standard or TRICARE Extra beneficiary, your annual deductible and maximum out-of-pocket expense is calculated by fiscal year. See the Fiscal Year Beginning date in this section for the first date of the fiscal year. If you are a TRICARE Prime beneficiary, your maximum out-of-pocket expense is calculated by enrollment and fiscal year. See Enrollment Year Beginning date in this section for the first date of your enrollment year. (**Note:** the Enrollment Year Beginning will appear on your EOB only if you are enrolled in TRICARE Prime.)

Remarks—Explanations of the codes or numbers listed in the "See Remarks" section will appear here.

Toll-Free Telephone Number—If you have questions about your TRICARE explanation of benefits use this toll-free number.

Double billing and Over Billing

Keep a record of all bills. Check all bills carefully and challenge anything that you are not sure of.

You may file an appeal if a claim you submitted is denied or is paid at a lower rate than you believe is appropriate, or if your request for a referral or authorization of a particular service is denied.

Covered versus Noncovered Procedure

Never Assume Anything. Be informed about what is covered before accepting an appointment.

Catastrophic Caps

A "catastrophic cap" is the annual upper limit a family will have to pay for TRICARE Standard-covered services in any fiscal year. The catastrophic cap for families of active duty service members is $1,000. All others have a catastrophic cap of $3,000. The catastrophic cap applies only to allowable charges for covered services. The catastrophic cap does not apply to services that are not covered, or to the total amount of what nonparticipating providers may charge above the TAC.

7

Funding Support and Legal Issues

FINANCIAL AND LEGAL PLANNING FOR THE FUTURE

All families must make plans for the future (short- and long-range). Most families have at one time or another faced challenges. Some of the challenges may be associated with meeting the needs of the family member with special needs.

General Finances

Finances play a major role in a family's decision-making process. Current finances are important. The "Benefits and allowances" section below provides information on financial management and the Services' Financial Readiness Programs.

Federal Programs

A number of federal programs provide financial assistance to families. Some are limited to families with low income regardless of disabilities, and others provide assistance to families with special needs regardless of income. See Federal Programs Providing Financial Assistance, available at MilitaryHOME-FRONT (www.militaryhomefront.dod.mil) for a summary of federal government programs that provide financial assistance to individuals and families either directly by cash payments or indirectly through some other means.

Transition Planning

Families must plan for the time their children are no longer eligible for some services because of their age. Transition from the public school system is a major transition point for families. See Transition Planning, at Military-HOMEFRONT for information on changes in program eligibility (schools and federal programs) as the child gets older, and about the child's rights when he or she reaches the age of majority (18 in most states).

Financial Planning

Financial planning involves many complex, emotional issues, especially if a family has a member with disabilities. Challenging as it may be, future planning can provide some realistic goals for the support of the family member when the parent or caregiver is no longer able to care for him or her.

Guardianship

When a child has a severe impairment, families must plan for the time when they are no longer the child's legal guardian. In most states, that is the age of 18.

BENEFITS AND ALLOWANCES

The following are Frequently Asked Questions about Personal Financial Management benefits and allowances.

Q: Who is eligible to use the Personal Financial Management Program (PFMP)?

A: Per Department of Defense (DoD) policy, the branches of service are required to make personal financial management programs, financial planning, and financial counseling services available to service members and their families. Although not specifically stated in policy, DoD civilians and military retirees may also take advantage of the services offered through PFMP offices on installations.

Q: Who is eligible to receive financial counseling through Military OneSource and the Military and Family Life Consultants (MFLC) Program?

A: All service members (active, reserve, and National Guard), DoD civilians, and their family members may schedule and receive financial counseling services through Military OneSource or the MFLC Program.

Q: How much does this financial training and counseling cost?

A: Although financial planning services can be very expensive in the civilian world, the services offered through PFMP offices, Military OneSource, and the MFLC Program are free of charge. Service members, DoD civilians, and their family members seeking financial counseling through Military OneSource or the MFLC program may receive up to twelve counseling sessions per issue. For those unable to attend face-to-face counseling, Military OneSource arranges telephone and online consultations.

BRANCH SUPPORT SERVICES

- **Army**
  - o Army Emergency Relief (AER)—AER is a nonprofit organization that assists Soldiers and their family members by providing emergency financial assistance, when there is a valid need, in the form of interest-free loans, grants, or a combination of the two.
  - o Army National Guard Consumer Affairs and Financial Assistance— The Army National Guard program provides financial education for Soldiers, civilians, and their families through classes, training, or information. More information on available classes can be found through the National Guard Family Assistance Centers.
  - o Army OneSource Financial Readiness—Army OneSource is the website of Army Community Service (ACS), the organization that provides family programs and services to members of the Army. This website assists Soldiers, civilians, and their families by providing budgeting and planning calculators, links to information on retirement planning, and online financial training, as well as a link to an Internet application which creates a graphic display of a visitor's financial profile.
  - o Army Reserve Family Programs Online Financial Readiness—This website assists and educates Soldiers and their families by providing information on financial planning, financial readiness training, the Thrift Savings Plan (TSP), and taxes.
- **Marine Corps**
  - o Marine Corps Personal Financial Management—The Personal Financial Management Program provides eligible personnel with education, training, counseling, information, and referrals for personal financial issues.
  - o Marine Corps Financial Fitness Online Resource Center—This website provides interactive financial tools and information to assist Marines and their families in controlling their finances. Topics include: financial planning, savings and investing, banking, credit decisions, using credit cards wisely, applying for credit, managing debt, and a "financial fitness checkup" application.

o Navy-Marine Corps Relief Society (NMCRS)—NMCRS is a private, nonprofit organization that provides financial, educational, and other assistance to members of the Navy and Marine Corps, eligible family members, and survivors when a valid need exists. NMCRS provides interest-free loans and grants to Sailors, Marines, and their families to meet emergency financial needs. NMCRS also provides financial education services such as budgeting counseling.

- **Navy**
  o Navy Fleet and Family Support Center (FFSC) Personal Financial Management (PFM)—The PFM Program assists members of the Navy family by providing information, classes, training, and counseling to combat financial mismanagement, as well as pro-active training to prepare Sailors and their families for future financial challenges.
  o Navy-Marine Corps Relief Society (NMCRS)—NMCRS is a private, nonprofit organization that provides financial, educational, and other assistance to members of the Navy and Marine Corps, eligible family members, and survivors when a valid need exists. NMCRS provides interest-free loans and grants to Sailors, Marines, and their families to meet emergency financial needs. NMCRS also provides financial education services such as budgeting counseling.
- **Air Force**
  o Air Force Community—The Air Force Community website provides information and links on a number of financial readiness topics to include credit and money management, home and car buying, personal finance and investing, tax information, and emergency financial assistance.
  o Air Force Aid Society (AFAS)—AFAS is a private, nonprofit organization that provides emergency financial assistance to Airmen and their family members. AFAS provides grants and interest-free loans to Airmen and their families who demonstrate an emergency financial need for essential costs, such as basic living expenses, medical care, funeral expenses, respite care, vehicle repairs, assistance with other emergencies, pay/allotment problems, and assistance to surviving dependents.
  o Air Force Compensation Fact Sheet—This fact sheet provides information on the benefits, entitlements, and opportunities available in an Air Force career. The fact sheet also contains Web links associated with each topic providing additional valuable information.
- **Coast Guard**
  o Coast Guard Mutual Assistance (CGMA)—CGMA is a private, nonprofit organization that provides financial assistance to members of

the Coast Guard community during times of need. CGMA provides persons associated with the Coast Guard, who demonstrate a financial need, with interest-free loans, personal grants, and confidential financial counseling and referral services.

GUARDIANSHIP

Guardianship is a legal relationship between a competent adult and a person over the age of 18, whose disability causes incompetency (a ward). The disability may be caused by mental illness, developmental disability, age, accident or other causes. (National Guardianship Association)

The subject of guardianship for a disabled child who is now an adult is of concern to most parents. Parents who have a child with a disability often assume that they can continue to be the legal guardian during the child's entire life. Although it may be obvious to a parent that their child does not have the capacity to make informed decisions, legally an adult is presumed competent unless otherwise deemed incompetent after a competency proceeding. In other words, once the child reaches the age of 18, the parent is no longer the child's legal guardian regardless of a disability.

The act of giving reasoned and well-informed consent when making a decision may be beyond the child's ability. In order to protect them from unscrupulous individuals who may exploit their inability to make informed choices, it is necessary for families to familiarize themselves with the various legal options available to protect a disabled child in adulthood. (Tuberous Sclerosis Alliance)

The Tuberous Sclerosis Alliance provides important information about guardianship and various alternatives to guardianship that are generally available to individuals with disabilities.

NOTE: It is important for families to research whether guardianship obtained in one state is transferable to another. Guardianship is not transferable in all states and may require a family to re-establish when they move.

8

Advocacy

Apart from everything else you have to do for your child, there is one other role that can be critical—and that is the role of advocate. You may not already realize it, but in many ways you are already advocating—learning about your child and his or her condition, keeping records and correspondence, and making sure your child receives the health care and education that he or she is entitled to.

EFFECTIVE COMMUNICATION

Effective communication is the cornerstone of successful advocacy. It doesn't matter who you are interacting with—your child's teacher, a school administrator, or health professional—effective communication ensures you get your message across without any confusion.

When dealing with your child's care, it can be very emotional, but it is important to stay calm and collected and talk in an even and modulated way. It is also a good idea to maintain direct eye contact and adopt positive, open body language—signs that you are being reasonable and attentive to the other person's viewpoint.

Shouting and waving your arms about will likely alienate whoever you are speaking to, and if you get too emotional you will be unlikely to present your case very well.

Being polite to someone doesn't mean you have to agree with them. However, if you remain calm, focused, and pleasant, it is more likely that you can discuss your differences in an open manner, which is more likely to lead to a successful outcome.

Even if you expect a meeting to be contentious, try to set a positive tone. Make good use of your manners, your smile, and direct eye contact. If you want the others to be patient, prepared, and educated about your child's needs, you must set the standard.

If you do not understand what someone has said, or if it rubs you the wrong way, politely say, "Did I understand you to say that _____?" This can clear up a misunderstanding early on or help define an area of disagreement. Do not be embarrassed to ask for further explanations. It is a parent's job to understand as much as possible about their child's education and medical condition. Look for common ground and be sure the others in the room know you are trying to understand their point of view. Thank those who have been helpful.

Despite the frustration and anger you may feel if a situation concerning your child is not heading toward consensus, it is advantageous to remain calm. You do not want to be seen as unreasonable, inconsistent, or volatile. Angry outbursts will undermine your credibility and thus your ability to advocate well.

It can be very frustrating to attend meetings or appointments and not understand the "lingo" that accompanies medical and educational dialogue with specialists, teachers, and various experts. Do not hesitate to ask them to define names and acronyms that they may use that are foreign to you. It can be helpful to ask what something means, how to spell it, and in what context it applies to your child. Do not be afraid to take notes and write down terms that you want to read about or look up later after the meeting is concluded. Certain assessments and tests have unusual names, and parents are often expected to already know what those names mean. Do not be afraid to be very clear about needing clarification and elaboration on subjects that are unfamiliar that relate to your child's educational or medical needs. Try to show patience with these individuals because they may not realize your level of familiarity or lack thereof, with their respective area of specialty.

Letter Writing

You may need to write letters for several reasons such as to request copies of school records, to request a meeting, or to document a problem. Some people are very comfortable with this, but if you are not, the following are some tips for effective letter writing:

Use clear, everyday language.
Keep it brief.
State the purpose of the letter in the first paragraph.

Explain what action you would like to see.
Finish the letter politely.
Include contact information.

Remember that once the letter is mailed, there is no going back. If a letter is written when you are angry, wait several days before mailing it. You may be rightfully upset, but the expression of your anger may hurt your cause, namely, the education of your child.

If no reply is received after 2 weeks, write again and include a copy of the first letter. If this letter brings no response, go higher up the chain of command.

Consider sending any correspondence in a manner that guarantees you either proof of delivery, signature or confirmation of receipt.

GETTING ORGANIZED

Corresponding with health-care agencies and school systems generates a lot of paper. To complicate things further, military families relocate every few years, which means you must often navigate through a new school system. Also, with each move comes the possibility of lost paperwork. What is needed is a system for organizing this paperwork because it is crucial to your ability to effectively advocate for your child.

To avoid the frustration of searching for lost letters or records, it is a good idea to have a system for keeping track of papers concerning your child's disability. For those with only a few papers, this might be as simple as a folder in which to keep letters from the school; for others it will be several binders, one for educational information and another for medical information. With well-organized records, you will be empowered as you go into meetings concerning your child's health or education.

Before you begin to organize these files, give thought to your child's needs. Are they primarily physical or educational? How many agencies have individual records for your child? Make a list of people and agencies in order to request records if needed. If you have a child with special educational needs as well as frequent medical needs, consider starting files in two separate binders: medical and educational.

The Medical File

The first binder will be primarily for medical information. Organize the sections in the following way:

Phone log
Research and information on the child's disability
Copies of correspondence to TRICARE
Correspondence from TRICARE
Other insurance information
Important pages from medical and dental records
Immunizations

If you would like copies of medical records, request them from the military treatment facility. The first copy should be provided free of charge. The policy for receiving copies of records varies at different facilities, but your request should be made in writing, and you may be asked to wait as long as 6 weeks to receive copies of your records.

Educational File

In the second binder, keep information about your child's educational history. Write a letter to request a complete copy of your child's educational records. You may want to start a photo record of your child on or in this binder, adding a school picture as each year goes by. Label dividers and organize information the following way:

Phone log
Assessments/evaluations
IEPs
Discipline reports
Report cards/interim reports
Correspondence to school system
Correspondence from school system
Immunizations and pertinent health records
Contact information for service providers and agencies

Remember to copy all letters you send to the school and include them in your file. Consider using certified mail when corresponding with the school system so there will be no question about if and when the school received your mail. Do not underestimate the value of an accurate phone log. Follow up important conversations with a note (e.g., "Thank you for talking with me today about my daughter's education. I understand that you have agreed to (provide/change) by (date). Please let me know if my understanding is not accurate."). Keep your notes from IEP meetings in this file, as well as any school suspension slips or notes from the school. Keep all documents in chronological order.

MEDICAL ADVOCACY

As you adjust to the news that your child has a physical or educational diagnosis, you may feel overwhelmed. Many parents react by learning all they can about their child's condition. Begin by asking your child's doctor and other professionals who know your child any questions you may have. Write down questions as they occur to you during the day. Then, at the next appointment, your questions will be ready. A thorough understanding of your child's condition will help you become aware of what you can expect from your child.

It may be empowering to learn all you can, but don't become overwhelmed with new information. Take time to adjust to the emotional impact of a new diagnosis. Remember that the diagnosis is only part of who your child is.

Getting the Referral You Need

A referral may be needed for a specific type of therapy or for special equipment for your child. Do not assume your doctor is aware of the best way to word the request.

A wonderful resource is the STOMP list serve, www.stompproject.org. STOMP is a Parent Training and Information Center for military families providing support and advice to military parents whose children have special challenges. Here you can interact with parents who have already experienced much of what you are going through. They are happy to help.

Armed with this information, you and your doctor can write a referral in the way most likely to be approved. If a piece of durable equipment is needed for your child, work with your health-care provider to write a very thorough and complete description of how a piece of durable equipment is going to lessen the functional loss caused by the disability.

Appealing TRICARE Decisions

If an application for Extended Care Health Option (ECHO) or Extended Home Health Care (EHHC) has been denied, the letter of denial will include the specific information you need about whether or not the decision is eligible for appeal, and if so where to send the letter of appeal and what the time limitations are. The appeal process varies depending on the reason for the denial. Even if the letter says the decision is not eligible for appeal, you may want to question it any way. Does the letter state the reason for the denial? Is it accurate? Can your child's circumstances be described in such a way as to make things more clear to TRICARE?

If your letter of denial states that an appeal is not available, do not give up quite yet. Question your TRICARE regional contractor as to the reason for the denial. Post a description of your problem on STOMP, www.stompproject.org, and see how other families have handled similar situations.

For help with TRICARE appeals, contact your regional contractor by going to www.tricare.mil and clicking on the applicable TRICARE region. You can also contact the Beneficiary Counseling and Assistance Coordinator (BCAC) at the TRICARE regional office or military treatment facility.

EDUCATIONAL ADVOCACY

It is especially important that parents whose children have special needs be aware of the legislation that affects how their children are educated.

Legislation

IDEA is the special education legislation that guides school systems throughout the United States, its territories, and Department of Defense schools in the education of children with special needs. The purpose of the law is to ensure that all children with disabilities have access to a free appropriate public education (FAPE), to ensure the rights of children with disabilities and those of their parents are protected, and to ensure that teachers and parents have the tools they need to meet educational goals and to assess the effectiveness of educational efforts being made for the child.

Section 504 of the Rehabilitation Act is a civil rights law that prohibits discrimination on the basis of disability and applies to public schools as well as employers or organizations that receive financial assistance from any federal department or agency. These organizations and employers include many hospitals, nursing homes, mental health centers, and human service programs. Because Section 504's definition of disability is broader than IDEA's definition, some children who do not qualify for special education under IDEA do qualify for special help under Section 504. This can be especially useful for children with "invisible" conditions, such as learning disabilities or Attention Deficit Hyperactivity Disorder. For more information about Section 504 of the Rehabilitation Act go to www.ed.gov.

The Americans with Disabilities Act (ADA) gives civil rights protection to individuals with disabilities similar to those provided to individuals on the basis of race, color, sex, national origin, age, and religion. It guarantees equal opportunity for individuals with disabilities in public accommodations, employment, transportation, state and local government services, and telecommunications. For more information about the ADA, visit www.usdoj.gov.

Nondiscrimination on the Basis of Handicap in Programs and Activities Assisted or Conducted by the Department of Defense, DoD Directive 1020.1, prohibits discrimination based on handicap in programs and activities receiving federal funds through the Department of Defense. For more information about this directive, go to www.dtic.mil.

For further information or assistance contact your state's Protection and Advocacy Agency. The National Disability Rights network lists state agencies at www.napas.org.

The School System

One of the basic principles of IDEA is that procedural safeguards must be in place to ensure that the rights of children and their parents are protected and that there are clear steps to follow in the case of a dispute. Contact your school system for information concerning appeals within the system. Ask for copies of these policies and procedures and take a well-read copy with you to your meetings. This will signal to the school that you are serious about your child's education, and that you know the rules. It is a good idea to contact your state Parent Training and Information Center and Community Parent Resource Centers. To find yours, contact Technical Assistance Alliance for Parent Training Centers, www.taalliance.org.

Assessments

A variety of tools may be used to help you and the school system identify your child's areas of strength and weakness. These often include IQ (or cognitive) tests or academic achievement tests given to your child in order to better define your child's intelligence or level of academic achievement. In either of these types of tests, a series of tasks are presented to the child being evaluated, and the child's responses are graded according to carefully prescribed guidelines. After the test is completed, the results are compiled and compared to the responses from other children of the same age or grade level as the child being evaluated. There are many assessments used, several are described below.

Differential Ability Scales (DAS). This a nationally normed and individually administered group of cognitive and achievement tests. Its age range includes children from 2 years and 6 months to 17 years and 11 months.

Leiter International Performance Scale. This is a totally nonverbal test of intelligence and cognitive abilities. It easily administered and quickly and objectively scored. Its game-like administration holds a child's interest.

Peabody Individual Achievement Test (PIAT). This is an efficient individual measure of academic achievement. Reading, mathematics, and spelling are assessed in a simple, nonthreatening format that requires only a pointing response for most items.

Stanford-Binet Intelligence Scales. This measures several types of reasoning, knowledge, and memory, testing both verbally and nonverbally in order to accurately assess individuals with deafness, limited English, or communication disorders.

Wechsler Intelligence Scale (WISC). This is an intelligence test for children between the ages of 6 and 16 that can be completed without reading or writing.

Woodcock-Johnson III (WJ III). This consists of two distinct batteries. Together they provide a comprehensive system for measuring general intellectual ability.

Speech and Language Tests

Speech and language issues are not separate from academic concerns, as speech and language form the basis for a child's ability to understand what is heard and to respond meaningfully. Children who have difficulty expressing themselves with spoken words may have difficulty putting their thoughts into words on paper. There are many tests that can assess whether your child has trouble with receptive language (understanding what is heard) or with expressive language (making oneself understood to others).

Understanding Scores

By examining your child's scores on norm-referenced tests, over time you will be able to gauge whether your child is attaining the goals or milestones with his peer group or falling behind. A criterion-referenced test can show if your child's score improves each year. However, if your child is steadily losing ground compared to peers, you may want to make some key changes to the IEP.

Grades given by teachers are an important piece of information, but may be quite subjective. Remember your teacher may give your child better grades than his or her work deserves out of kindness, as a reward for sincere effort, or because failing grades will increase the pressure on the teacher. For a clear picture of your child's progress, standardized norm-referenced tests are a good evaluation tool.

If there is a steady decline in your child's progress as compared to peers, and you believe that a more effective educational plan could change it, consider making a chart of your child's standardized test scores. Bring the chart to the next IEP meeting, as a visual image sometimes has more impact than spoken words.

The composite score is the combination of all subjects assessed and may be misleading, as it will not show variation between subjects. The composite score will not show you variation between subjects. Beware of looking only at composite scores from the battery of tests your child has taken. If you have a child with an obvious strength in one area and a weakness in another, the scores may blend into an average composite score that seems to show that your child is of average capability and offers no explanation for any educational frustration. If you look at the subtest scores you might see that your child has an area of weakness that is interfering with his or her education.

The bell curve and standard deviations. The bell curve is a visual way of organizing data, in this case test scores. The center of the bell, where it is the highest, shows the average test score, or the fiftieth percentile. Those who did better than the average score will fall to the right of center and those who did less than the average score will fall to the left. So, within the bell curve you will find the entire spectrum of scores of the population that was tested. As there are few children who do very well or very poorly, the size of the bell diminishes as it moves outward.

To describe how far a score falls from the center, or average, we use standard deviations. The phrase "standard deviation" refers to the distance between a certain score and the average score. The average score will be in the center of the bell at 0 standard deviations. The next markers move away from the center and are -1 and +1, -2 and+2, and -3 and +3. The percentage of scores that fall between the deviations is always the same, so that between -1 and +1 standard deviation is where 68% of the population will fall. In a normal distribution, about 68% of the scores are within one standard deviation of the mean and about 95% of the scores are within two standard deviations of the mean. So, if your child scored at the +1 standard deviation, she has scored at the 84th percentile.

Independent Educational Evaluations

Before an IEP or eligibility meeting, ask for copies of any new evaluations. If you think that the evaluation conducted by the school is either out of date or incomplete, you have several options. You may ask your school to re-administer a test, or have it administered by another person. If you are still dissatisfied, you can request an independent educational evaluation (IEE) of your child at public expense.

You do not have to prove that the school's evaluation was faulty. You are entitled to an independent evaluation if there is reason to believe the initial evaluation is incomplete or inaccurate. An IEE may evaluate any skill related to your child's educational needs. The school may not agree to this independent evaluation and may choose to hold a hearing during which they will try to show that the initial evaluation was valid and complete. Unless they do this, the school system cannot deny your request for a new evaluation. A sample letter requesting an independent evaluation can be found in chapter 10 of this book.

If, after a hearing, the school system is not required to pay for an independent educational evaluation, you may still choose to have your child evaluated independently at your own expense. Private evaluations are not cheap, but can be very useful. School district evaluations are school district material, and in the case of an independent hearing they are important evidence. You may be reassured the independent testing reinforces what the school system has found or dismayed that there is a discrepancy, but you need not question the veracity of the independent evaluation.

IEP and Eligibility Meetings

IEP and eligibility meetings can be emotionally laden. Even if you have a good relationship with your child's teachers and school system, learning that your child is lagging behind his or her peers can be a devastating blow. On the other hand, trying to convince the school system to provide services for your child when the school system is resistant can be profoundly frustrating as well. Keep the focus on your child, and not on the school district's resources or any individual personalities in the room. There may be tension between your wishes and expectations as a parent and the school district's resources. As a parent, you want the best for your child. But the school district must provide services from within a clearly stated budget.

If both parents cannot attend the IEP meeting, it is a good idea to bring a friend or family member who has experience with your child to the meeting. The moral support can be invaluable. Also, when the meeting is over it is very helpful to have someone who was there and who can offer a different perspective with whom you can discuss the meeting.

Writing an Effective IEP

To write an effective IEP, you must first have an accurate understanding of your child's present level of achievement and functional performance. By reviewing the assessments your child has taken, you will be able to see the areas of need that arise as a function of your child's disability. Have a clear idea of your ultimate goals for your child. What are the steps that your child must take to reach these goals? Think about the skills your child needs to progress. What does your child need to learn? Does your child need to learn to communicate, to get along with peers, or to read?

A good IEP will specifically identify the following:

Areas where growth is needed
Activities and services the child will receive to help encourage growth and
    learning
How often your child will participate in these activities and where
How your child's progress will be measured, and at what intervals

A well-constructed IEP will state goals and objectives that are well defined and measurable. "Joey will improve his reading and skills" is not specific, does not give a time limit, and does not tell us how the improvement will be measured. Better would be an IEP that states, "In six months time, Joey will increase reading skills to the third grade level, as measured by . . . "

Disagreements

If presented with an IEP that was completed before the meeting began, keep in mind that you have a right to participate in the development of your child's IEP. Consider and refer to this IEP as a draft. If you feel pressured to sign it, simply remind the other members of the committee that you need time to read and digest such an important document, and you will need a copy to take home with you.

If you have serious concerns about the IEP, put them in writing and return them to the school along with the unsigned IEP. You may want to request another IEP meeting. Remember that your child cannot begin to receive services until you have given permission. If necessary, you can agree in writing to part of the IEP, but not all. This way your child can begin to receive the agreed-upon services.

It may happen that the meeting ends before you have finished the IEP. The school may ask you to sign this. You are taking a risk if you sign an unfinished document. Consider saying you are not ready to sign such an important document yet and would like to wait until it is completed and then read it before signing it.

Should any of these disagreements occur, you may request an administrative review within the school system. If this is not available or the results are not satisfactory, you have two options: mediation or due process.

Mediation is a process that resolves disputes without litigation. When you mediate, you have two goals: to resolve the dispute and to protect your relationship with the school system.

Due process hearings are conducted differently from state to state; however, they provide an opportunity to have your complaint heard in an impartial hearing. Before the hearing takes place, the school must hold a Resolution Session to give the parties a chance to resolve their differences before the hearing.

You may request mediation or a due process hearing, or you may request both at the same time. This will accelerate the process and lessen the amount of time your child must wait for an appropriate education. Your state Parent Training Center (www.taalliance.org) can help.

If you are involved with a DoD school, you can find the details about your rights in DoDI 1342.12, the Provision of Early Intervention and Special Education Services to Eligible DoD Dependents (www.dtic.mil).

Even if you are considering it, avoid threatening to ask for a due process hearing. The school has heard this many times before, and the threat is unlikely to have the effect you hope for. Also, on further reflection you may decide you do not want to file for due process after all.

BENEFITS ADVOCACY

In addition to the benefits available to military families, there are also federal and state benefits that your child may be eligible for.

Supplemental Security Income (SSI)

SSI is a monthly payment to those with low incomes and few resources who are 65 or older, blind, or disabled. Children may qualify. If you think you or your child might qualify, visit your nearest Social Security Office or call the Social Security Administration Office at 1-800-772-1213. If your application is denied, it is good practice to appeal the decision. Keep in mind that the appeal should be timely, no later than 30 days from the date of the notice or 10 days if you are requesting to receive benefits during the appeal. This is referred to as "aid paid pending." Be aware that you may be asked to repay the benefits if the outcome is not in your favor. Also, as you move from state to state you will find that eligibility requirements vary.

Medicaid

Medicaid is a program that pays for health care for some individuals and families with low income and few resources. Medicaid is a national program with broad guidelines, but each state sets its own eligibility rules and decides what services to provide. Be aware of this as you move from state to state. States can also choose to cover other groups of children under the age of 19 or those who live in higher-income families.

Many states qualify children through a program called TEFRA (Tax Equity and Fiscal Responsibility Act of 1982, also known as the Katie Beckett Waiver) or the Home and Community Based Waiver. These programs allow children to qualify without considering their parents' income. To find information on Medicaid and Medicaid waivers in your state go to www.cms.hhs.gov.

Military families who are struggling with the cost of care for a disabled family member should consider applying for Medicaid. Benefits may exceed those offered by TRICARE.

To apply, contact www.cms.hhs.gov/medicaid.

TEACHING YOUR CHILD TO SELF-ADVOCATE

As a parent you know how important it is to teach your child as much as possible about taking care of himself or herself. This may mean teaching personal hygiene, how to safely cross a street, or how to avoid a classmate who always causes trouble. Teaching self-advocacy is not very different. If we expect our children to grow as people, we must give them the chance to speak for themselves and to make their own decisions.

Self-advocacy begins with teaching your child to ask for help and to accept responsibility for his or her own actions. Part of this is being an active participant in planning his or her life. It means helping your child feel confident enough to speak out when something is bothering him or her. This can be practiced at home or at school. Self-advocacy can take many forms, such as explaining to a new teacher the need to tape record the lesson, informing the waiter that he made a mistake on the order, or learning to use public transportation. It can begin with letting your child pay for purchases or plan a birthday party. It is very important for students with disabilities to develop or improve self-advocacy skills because they will need these skills in all life settings.

The transition process at your child's school can help. Transition is when the focus of your child's education begins to shift from identifying and working to minimize your child's challenges to looking toward the future and exploring what it will take for your child to learn a job or live on his or her own. Your student should be an integral part of this process, expressing needs, wants, and desires. To have a full life, your child must be part of the plan.

One of the most adult services, vocational rehabilitation, is available through your state. Vocational rehabilitation services include planning, assistance, support, and training to help disabled people get ready for and find a job. Most states have a vocational rehabilitation agency with regional offices that provide these services. If you know you will retire in a different state, contact them. Remember that waiting lists for assisted living homes can be years long. Contact your state Parent Training Center (www.taalliance.org) to find out what programs are available in your state.

INFLUENCING PUBLIC LAW

With day-to-day life as full as it is, keeping track of new and proposed legislation may be low on your list of things to do; however, you have the power to influence the legislation that will impact your child's education, health, and quality of life.

What can a busy parent do? The first step is to be informed. Many parents find list serves a place to not only share tips on how to get through the day, but also a place to become informed about public issues that may affect their child. Your state Parent Training Center is another source to ask about current issues.

When an issue of importance to you comes up, a quick phone call or a one-page letter to an elected official's office is all it takes to express a view. Elected officials pay attention to communications from constituents. Tell your family's story. If you are sending a letter or an e-mail, include a picture of your family. This will put a face on the issue at hand for your representative, who will likely know the details of the legislation but may need to hear about how it will affect the lives of his or her constituents.

Parents can share personal stories about what public education and other health government services have done for their family. In addition, they can explain about their need for additional services and funding.

Seek Other Parents of Children with Disabilities

The Exceptional Family Member Representative can help you find other families who have faced similar challenges. The knowledge that you are not alone can be of great comfort. Find your EFMP representative through your Family Service Center.

Also available through Military Homefront is the Family Connections Forum at www.militaryhomefront.dod.mil.

Contact STOMP

Specialized Training of Military Parents (STOMP) is a valuable resource. They provide support and advice to military parents without regard to the type of medical or educational condition the child may have. STOMP also has many excellent publications on their website. You can join their list serve and correspond with other parents of specially challenged children. Go to www.stompproject.org or call 1-800-5-parent.

Find Your State Parent Training and Information Center

Each state is home to at least one parent center (www.taalliance.org/centers). Parent centers serve families of children and young adults from birth to age 22 with all disabilities: physical, cognitive, emotional, and learning. They help families obtain appropriate education and services for their children with disabilities; work to improve education results for all children; train and inform parents and professionals on a variety of topics; resolve problems between families and schools or other agencies; and connect children with disabilities to community resources that address their needs.

BOOKS

From Emotions to Advocacy, second edition, by Pam and Pete Wright (This is an excellent source for advocacy information.)

Writing Measurable IEP Goals and Objectives, by Barbara D. Bateman and Cynthia M. Herr

The Goal Mine: Nuggets of Learning Goals and Objectives for Exceptional Children, (Paperback) by Donald Cahill, Maureen Cahill

How Well Does Your IEP Measure Up? Quality Indicators for Effective Service Delivery, by Dianne Twachtman-Cullen and Jennifer Twachtman-Reilly, with foreword by David L. Holmes, Ed.D.

The Complete IEP Guide, 4th Edition: How to Advocate for Your Special Ed Child, by attorney Lawrence M. Siegel

EP Magazine, www.eparent.com

9

Coping

ROLLER COASTER OF EMOTIONS

When parents recognize their child is not going to have a typical course of development into adulthood, their lives are changed forever. At best, they experience a roller coaster of emotions that include the initial shock and sadness of learning their child has special needs, to fear of the responsibility of caring for them, to anger and frustration as they negotiate complex systems trying to get the special needs met. These painful emotions are, of course, intertwined with intense love and admiration for their child's unique qualities as a human being and pride in his or her accomplishments. At worst, parents of special needs children allow themselves to be defined by their children's circumstances. These parents may suffer significant depression or intense anger at their child, spouse, or others in their environment. Where a parent is on this emotional continuum is influenced by his or her personality style and coping skills, the family's strength and unity, and the support and encouragement available from others.

Most special needs parents develop a sense of confidence, resiliency, and determination as a consequence of the demands of parenting a disabled child. Yet nearly every one of them, at certain times, will need help in developing the skills necessary to cope with parenting a special needs child and in managing the emotions that emerge. A few of them will need specific interventions to help them avoid the risk of abuse or neglect. This section offers options that may be suggested to parents who are in need of support as well as services for those at risk.

Counseling

Counseling is a way for people who are facing situations or emotions that they feel they can't handle or control to find help from a trained professional. A counselor will listen to the problem and ask probing questions to get at a deeper level of what is going on and then either explore with the client ways to change his or her thinking about an issue or teach skills that can be used to better manage feelings or situations. Counseling to help someone deal with a stressful or painful situation may require only a few sessions. By contrast, individuals who have serious emotional difficulties that are not in response to an immediate set of circumstances will need psychiatric care in which counseling may be just one component. Parents of EFMs should be referred for counseling if they seem to be having difficulty accepting the child and coping with his/her needs or if they are feeling overwhelming emotions. Military parents have several options for cost-free counseling.

Military OneSource

One of the benefits of Military OneSource is that it offers twelve free in-person counseling sessions per person, per issue. For those unable to attend face-to-face counseling, Military OneSource arranges telephone and online consultations. Military ID card holders can be referred to a counselor in their area who is part of Military OneSource's extensive network of licensed and credentialed professionals. A call to the toll-free number, 1-800-655-4545 is the first step in being connected with a counseling professional.

Chaplains/Ministers

Many people are more comfortable seeking counseling that has a spiritual component. When parents of EFMs seem to be having difficulty coping, it is good to ask them about their religious ties before making a referral for counseling. Military chaplains and ministers in the civilian community often have professional counseling expertise over and above their ability to provide spiritual guidance and support.

Family Centers

Family Centers have been one of the strongest strands in the network of community services available at military installations for active duty personnel and their families. For the past 25 years, Family Centers have been the primary resource for information, direct services, and support for families as they coped with the unique challenges of the military lifestyle. Today, there is a new source of assistance for service members and their families regardless of where they may be located around the world. Special needs families should know about both options.

Some military family centers offer short-term, solution-focused counseling within their programs. At the very least, family centers will provide consultation, assessment, and referral for counseling, plus help arrange respite care, if necessary, during counseling sessions. Use MilitaryHOMEFRONT's MilitaryINSTALLATIONS Directory to locate a Family Center near you.

Note: Anytime a person expresses the desire or intention to hurt his- or herself or others, immediate action should be taken to ensure an emergency evaluation at a medical treatment facility. Counseling will be needed later after the person has stabilized emotionally.

Peer Support

Many people caring for a disabled family member have found emotional support through relationships with other parents in similar situations. Talking to others who share the same experiences, emotions, and concerns can be extremely reassuring as well as a source of new skills, knowledge, and insight. Opportunities for peer support can be in person, through organized groups dealing with a particular issue or condition, and in cyberspace through online discussion groups, chats, and list serves.

Support Groups

Many installation family centers sponsor or have information on support groups for military special needs families. Local hospitals and schools often organize support groups around a particular disability, such as autism. Support groups may also be located by contacting the national association for a particular disability.

Parent-to-Parent Programs

These programs are organized at the state and local levels to offer support and information to parents of children with disability, chronic illness, or special needs. A typical parent-to-parent program will match a "support parent"—a trained volunteer who has developed effective coping skills and strategies for parenting a child with special needs—with a "referred parent" who has a child newly diagnosed, in crisis, in transition, or simply in need of support. Parents are matched as closely as possible based on the child's diagnosis, family structure, and ethnic or religious similarities. The kind, frequency, and duration of contacts vary based on individual needs. The Beach Center on Disability at the University of Kansas maintains an updated list of links to Parent-to-Parent groups by state.

Online Chat, Discussion Boards, and List Serves

Parents of special needs children are increasingly turning to the Internet to find support and encouragement. Many national associations for specific disabilities sponsor online discussion groups. The Specialized Training of Military Parents (STOMP) has a list serve for military special needs families.

PERSONAL FORTITUDE

It is amazing how strong and resilient one can be when one has to be. Caring for and coping with a special needs child is a 24/7 job but, as all parents of special needs children know, it can be thoroughly rewarding.

Of course, it is tiring and stressful, and dealing with all the paperwork and officials can be tedious and frustrating, but the information in this book is aimed at helping you cope with that.

It is important to always remember that you are not alone—even if sometimes you think you are. There is always someone you can turn to for support and help either on the installation or in the neighboring community. We have included the names of hundreds of organizations whose sole purpose is to help people like you.

You need to be strong as a caregiver, and that means looking after yourself. You need to be aware of the signs of "caregiver stress" and what you can do to mitigate or prevent this.

Signs include:

- **Emotional warning signs:**
    o Anger
    o Inability to concentrate
    o Unproductive worry
    o Sadness and periodic crying
    o Frequent mood swings
- **Physical warning signs:**
    o Stooped posture
    o Sweaty palms
    o Tension headaches

o Neck pain
o Chronic back pain
o Chronic fatigue
o Weight gain or loss
o Problems with sleep
- **Behavioral warning signs**
  o Overreacting
  o Acting on impulse
  o Using alcohol or drugs
  o Withdrawing from relationships
  o Changing jobs often

Tips for managing stress include:

Keep a positive attitude. Believe in yourself.

Accept that there are events you cannot control.

Be assertive instead of aggressive. "Assert" your feelings, opinions, or beliefs instead of becoming angry, combative, or passive.

Learn to relax.

Exercise regularly. Your body can fight stress better when it is fit.

Stop smoking.

Limit yourself to moderate alcohol and caffeine intake.

Set realistic goals and expectations.

Get enough rest and sleep. Your body needs time to recover from stressful events.

Don't rely on alcohol or drugs to reduce stress.

Learn to use stress management techniques and coping mechanisms, such as deep breathing or guided imagery.

If you don't look after yourself, you will not be able to look after anyone else. Eat well, sleep well, exercise often, and take time for an occasional time-out.

RESOURCEFULNESS

Looking after a child with special needs automatically means you are resourceful—you have to be. It is that resourcefulness that drives you to do what's best for your child and that means knowing what's best for him or her. You have to familiarize yourself with all the laws and regulations, educational requirements, and medical procedures so that you can be the best possible advocate for your child. Having that knowledge will empower and give you tremendous confidence facing the challenges along the way.

If you are religious your faith will also give you additional comfort and strength and the support of your extended church family. You also have the support of your own family and friends and the much larger military family to which you belong.

With all this support surrounding you, you should never be alone—or feel alone. Never be afraid to ask for help—it is all around you and only minutes away.

Being a caregiver with a special needs child is one of the most challenging jobs there is and one of the most important. However, there is nothing more rewarding.

10

Resources

SAMPLE LETTERS

When caring for your child, it might be difficult to take the time to consider that, at some point, illness may prevent you from continuing to provide that care. It is even harder to consider that your child may outlive you. You have provided a level of care that you would want to ensure continued. You would not want your child's quality of life to be affected or altered in any significant way, and you would not want his or her brothers or sisters to be solely responsible for providing care.

While the entire SCOR can be considered a letter of intent, this section is focused on helping you organize information and plans in the event that someone would have to take over caring for your child. It can be used to facilitate discussion among your family members or to organize your own thoughts. Identifying a guardian can be one of the most emotional and difficult decisions to tackle. It might be helpful to talk to an attorney at your installation's legal assistance office for a referral to a civilian attorney who specializes in setting up guardianships and in creating special needs trusts.

Although some of the material in this section might seem daunting, take the time to go through each page and organize your thoughts. Completing these pages can help ensure that your child continues to receive the level of care that you want him or her to have into the future.

SAMPLE LETTER REQUESTING AN EVALUATION

Your Address
Your Phone Number
Date

Special Education Director or Program Coordinator
School District
Street Address
City, State, Zip

Dear _____:
I am requesting a complete evaluation for my son/daughter (Name, date of birth) to determine if my child qualifies as a special education student as stipulated in the Individuals with Disabilities Education Act (IDEA), P.L. 105-17, Section 614 (a)–(c).

I understand that the evaluation is to be provided at no charge to me. My reasons for requesting this procedure are _____.

I would appreciate meeting with each person who will be doing the evaluation prior to testing my child so that I might share information about (child's name) with him/her. I will also expect a copy of the written report generated by each evaluator so that I might review it before the team meeting.

I understand that I have to give written permission for these tests to be administered and I will be happy to do so upon receipt of the proper forms.

I appreciate your help in this matter. If you have any questions, please call me at (telephone number).

Sincerely,
Your signature
Your Name typed
cc: Principal
District Superintendent

Sample Letter Requesting a Reevaluation

Your Name
Address
Phone Number

Date

Special Education Director or Program Coordinator
School District
Street Address
City, State, Zip

Dear _____:
We are requesting a total evaluation of our son/daughter, (Name), birth date _____, under P.L. 105-17, Section 614 (c). We understand that this testing process will be done in compliance with (cite appropriate sections of state regulations).
We are requesting this re-evaluation because

_____

_____.

We understand that we will be a part of the team that will determine the evaluations that are needed and that we will be required to provide permission to do the re-assessment.

We will be happy to sign the necessary paperwork when it is provided. We also understand that we will receive a copy of the results of the re-assessment, and look forward to getting those results.

We appreciate your help and will be expecting to hear from you soon regarding the re-evaluation.

Sincerely,
Your signature
Your Name typed
cc: Principal
District Superintendent

Sample Letter Requesting an Independent Evaluation

Your Name
Address
Your Phone Number
Date

Special Education Director or Program Coordinator

School District
Street Address
City, State, Zip

Dear _____:

I am requesting an independent assessment at public expense for my son/ daughter, (Name), birth date, _____. This request is made pursuant to P.L. 105-17, Section 614 (a)–(c).

I am requesting this independent assessment in the area of (stipulate academics, speech, occupational therapy, physical therapy, vocational or vision therapy). I am requesting this independent assessment because I do not agree with the district results in this area. (Explain briefly with what you disagree; e.g., not accurate, no test available in the district, not complete, etc).

I understand that a response to my request must be provided in writing by the school district within ten (10) days.

I appreciate your help. If you have any questions, please call me at (telephone number).

Sincerely,
Your signature
Your Name typed
cc: Principal
District Superintendent

Sample Letter Requesting a Records Review

Your Name
Address
Your Phone Number
Date

Special Education Director or Program Coordinator
School District
Street Address
City, State, Zip

Dear _____:

I would like to review any and all educational records held in any form and in any location by _____ School District for my son/daughter, (Name), birth date. This request is made pursuant to P.L. 105-17, Section 615 (b).

I understand that someone will be available to answer any questions I may have regarding my son's/daughter's school records.

I look forward to meeting with you in the near future. If you have any questions, please call me at (telephone number).

Sincerely,
Your signature
Your Name typed
cc: Principal
District Superintendent

Sample Letter Requesting a Correction or Removal of Information Contained in Records

Your Name
Address
Your Phone Number
Date

Special Education Director or Program Coordinator
School District
Street Address
City, State, Zip

Dear _____:

Upon review of my son's/daughter's, (Name), birth date, _____, records, I find a need to request that _____ School District remove or correct the information dealing with (give specific area) found in (give document, date and person responsible for document; e.g., psychological evaluation dated 6-7-97 by Dr. Paul Doe). I am making this request pursuant to P.L. 105-17, Section 615 (b).

I will be expecting to hear from you within five (5) working days regarding this matter.

Thank you.

Sincerely,
Your signature
Your Name typed
cc: Principal
   District Superintendent

Sample Letter Requesting a Due Process Hearing

Your Name
Address
Your Phone Number
Date

(This letter must be sent to either the superintendent of the public school your child attends, or to the State Department of Education, whichever is specified by your state:)
Street Address
City, State, Zip

Dear _____:

We are requesting a due process hearing as stipulated in P.L. 105-17, Section 615 (e) and (f).

This request is made by us on behalf of our son/daughter, (Name), birth date _____, (child's address, if different than yours), who attends _____ school within _____School District.

We are requesting this due process hearing because

_____
_____
_____.

To the best of our knowledge at this time, we feel the district should (describe here any possible solutions you feel would alleviate the problem).

Since the district and we are unable to find resolution for this/these problem(s), we find it necessary to move forward with our procedural rights. We are willing to participate in a mediation hearing as a part of this process, but understand that it will not delay or deny us our right to due process. We are also willing to meet with a hearing officer in a pre-hearing conference.

We would like a list of any free or low-cost legal/advocacy help available, a copy of our due process rights, and a list of hearing officers and their qualifications.

We regret that we have had to come to this method of resolution, but feel it necessary. We expect to hear from you soon.

Sincerely,
Your signature
Your Name typed

cc: Principal
Special Education Director
Attorney

Sample Letter Regarding Suspension of a Student with a Disability (not related to weapons or drugs)

Your Name
Address
Your Phone Number
Date

Special Education Director or Program Coordinator
School District
Street Address
City, State, Zip

Dear _____:

We have been notified that our son/daughter, (Name), birth date _____, has been suspended for (number of days) from (school name- school district). We are notifying you of our understanding of procedures that must be conducted in compliance with P.L. 105-17, Section 615 (k), the Individuals with Disabilities Education Act (IDEA).

Our child has an Individual Education Program (IEP) and we understand that because he/she receives special education services, a meeting must be held no later than 10 school days after a decision to suspend/expel has been made, or immediately if the cumulative total of suspensions total 10 school days. We understand that the purpose of this meeting will be to determine if the reason for the suspension is related to his/her disability and to discuss his/her IEP goals and objectives, placement, and determine if a functional behavioral assessment is needed. We also understand that the number of days he/she can be suspended is not to exceed ten (10) cumulative school days in a given year, without notice of change of placement and all due process procedures, since he/she is in special education. Additionally, it is our understanding that the school district remains responsible for providing appropriate educational and related services, as outlined in his/her current IEP to include access to the general education curriculum, during the period of suspension.

We would like to meet with you as soon as possible to discuss this. Please call us at (telephone number).

Sincerely,
Your signature
Your Name typed

cc: School District Superintendent

Sample Letter Regarding Suspension and Expulsion When Weapons or Drugs are Involved

Your Name
Address
Your Phone Number
Date

Superintendent of School District
School District
Street Address
City, State, Zip

Dear _____:

We are writing in response to the notice that our son/daughter has been unilaterally placed into an interim alternative placement for weapon/drug violations in compliance with P.L. 105-17, Section 615 (k) (1) (A) (ii) of the Individuals with Disabilities Education Act (IDEA).

We understand that a Manifestation Determination meeting will be scheduled within the next 10 school days to determine if the behavior is related to the disability. We also understand that we will have the opportunity to be a part of the decision-making team regarding the interim alternative placement and the provision of services. As this placement will be for up to 45 calendar days, we feel it is important that (child's name) program, as currently outlined in his/her IEP, be followed, and that he/she have access to the general education curriculum, although in a different setting.

We are requesting a copy of all of our procedural due process rights. Please contact us as quickly as possible regarding the meeting to determine if this is or is not a manifestation and to talk about the interim alternative placement.

We appreciate your assistance during this difficult situation. If you have any questions, please feel free to contact us at (telephone number).

Sincerely,
Your signature
Your Name typed

cc: Principal

Sample Letter Requesting an Expedited Due Process Hearing

Your Name
Address
Your Phone Number
Date

(This letter must be sent to either the Superintendent of the public school your child attends, or to the State Department of Education, whichever is specified by your state.)
Street Address
City, State, Zip

Dear _____ :

We are requesting an expedited due process hearing as stipulated in P.L. 105-17, Section 615 (k) (6) (A). This request is made by us on behalf of our son/daughter, (Name), birth date _____, (child's address, if different than yours), who attends _____ school within _____ School District.

We are making this request because we disagree with the determination that (your child's name) behavior was not a manifestation of his/her disability, *or*, the decision regarding placement of (your child's name) made because of the discipline procedures. Our reasons for this disagreement are

_____

_____

_____.

At this time we feel it is necessary for (name of school district) to (state here any solution you feel would be necessary to resolve this problem, to the extent you know a solution at this time).

We understand that you will be contacting us shortly regarding the date, place, and time of this expedited hearing. We understand that an impartial hearing officer, from the pool of hearing officers for special education hearings, will preside over this hearing.

We are requesting a copy of our procedural safeguards as part of this request. We appreciate your expedient response to our request.

Sincerely,
Your signature
Your Name typed

cc: Principal
Special Education Director

Sample Letter Documenting a Telephone Call

Your Name
Address
Your Phone Number
Date

(Name)
Title
Street Address
City, State, Zip

Dear _____:

Thank you for talking with me today on the telephone. I appreciate your concern for (child's name). I understand from our conversation that you are

concerned about, OR, As I mentioned on the telephone I am concerned about
_____.

    You feel _____ will help and the
school has agreed to _____. I also said that I
would_____.

    Thank you for your help. If you have any questions, please call me at
(telephone number).

    Sincerely,
    Your signature
    Your Name typed

Sample Letter Documenting a Meeting

    Your Name
    Address
    Your Phone Number
    Date

    (Name)
    Title
    Street Address
    City, State, Zip

Dear _____:
Thank you for taking the time to meet with me on (date). Also,
please thank (list names) for attending the meeting. I understand that
you are concerned about _____. OR, As I reported during the
meeting, I am concerned about _____. You
feel _____ will help and the school has agreed to
_____. I also said that I would _____
_____.

    Thank you for your help. If you have any questions, please call me at
(telephone number).

    Sincerely,
    Your signature
    Your Name typed

TRANSITIONING A SPECIAL NEEDS STUDENT CHECKLIST

Before you leave your current duty station:

_____ Contact your local EFMP Manager or School Liaison Officer for assistance.

_____ Schedule an Annual Review and Dismissal (ARD) meeting to discuss the progress your child has made since your last Individualized Education Program (IEP) review. Ask for written suggestions that may help your child and the staff at the new school.

_____ Request a copy of your child's complete educational record to include a copy of the latest IEP. **Hand carry** all records, samples of your child's work, and other information related to your child's education to the new school.

_____ If the EFMP Manager at the new duty station doesn't contact you, make sure you contact them. They can assist you with identifying resources at your new duty station.

_____ Be sure to take any special equipment and refill medication prescriptions that your child may need for the next few months.

RED CROSS LINKS

Both active duty and community-based military can count on the Red Cross to provide emergency communications that link them with their families back home, access to financial assistance from the military aid societies, counseling, referral to community resources, and assistance to veterans. Red Cross Service to the Armed Forces (SAF) personnel form a global network in more than 700 U.S. chapters, 58 military installations worldwide, and in forward-deployed locations in Kuwait, Afghanistan, and Iraq.

- **Military Members and Families**—www.redcross.org/services/afes/0,1082,0_321_,00.html
- **Emergency Communication Services**—www.redcross.org/services/afes/0,1082,0_476_,00.html
- **Emergency Financial Assistance**—www.redcross.org/services/afes/0,1082,0_477_,00.html
- **Counseling**—www.redcross.org/services/afes/0,1082,0_478_,00.html
- **Services for Veterans**—www.redcross.org/services/afes/0,1082,0_479_,00.html
- **Active Duty Military Personnel**—www.redcross.org/services/afes/0,1082,0_480_,00.html

- **Reserves and National Guard**—www.redcross.org/services/afes/0,1082,0_481_,00.html
- **Deployment Tips**—www.redcross.org/services/afes/0,1082,0_482_,00.html
- **Military/Red Cross Partnership**—www.redcross.org/services/afes/0,1082,0_484_,00.html
- **Military Members and Families FAQs**—www.redcross.org/faq/0,1095,0_380_,00.html

INTERNET LINKS

Transition Services

Transition Assistance Program—The official transition assistance website, operated under contract on behalf of U.S. Department of Defense, U.S. Department of Labor, and U.S. Department of Veterans Affairs. www.transitionassistanceprogram.com/register.tpp

U.S. Dept of Labor Transition Assistance Program (TAP) Information—www.dol.gov/vets/programs/tap/

Housing Transition—The VA offers help in locating available services for temporary housing and other associated services. See www.va.gov/homeless/ to review VA resources.

Women Veterans Comprehensive Health Center—www.va.gov/wvhp/

National Coalition for Homeless Veterans—nchv.org/

Military Transition Programs

U.S. Army Wounded Warrior Program—aw2portal.com/Default.aspx

U.S. Marine Corps Wounded Warrior Regiment (WWR)—www.manpower.usmc.mil/pls/portal/url/page/m_ra_home/wwr

U.S. Air Force Palace HART Program—www.af.mil/news/story.asp?id=123020008 (news story, 5/5/2006)

U.S. Navy Safe Harbor Program—www.npc.navy.mil/CommandSupport/SafeHarbor

Disability Information for Veterans and the Military Community—www.disabilityinfo.gov/digov-public/public/DisplayPage.do?parentFolderId=179

Support Agencies for Wounded Service Members, Wounded Families—www.militarymoney.com/home/1140115165/

Resources for Wounded or Injured Service members and Their Families—www.nmfa.org/site/DocServer/Wounded_Servicemember7-06.pdf?docID=6703 (National Military Family Association Fact Sheet)

Employment Information

Department of Veterans Affairs Job Information—The U.S. Department of Veterans Affairs is always seeking to hire disabled veterans and veterans of all eras. To view the latest information on job openings in VA and how to apply please visit the **VA Jobs** site. www.va.gov/jobs/

U.S. Department of Labor Veterans' Employment and Training Service (VETS)—DOL is charged with job and job training counseling service, employment placement service, and job training placement service for eligible veterans as carried as out by the Department of Labor. www.dol.gov/vets/programs/empserv/

Vet Success—The purpose of the **vetsuccess.gov** site is to present information about the VA Vocational Rehabilitation and Employment (VR&E) Program provided to veterans with service-connected disabilities. It also provides information about vocational counseling available to active duty service members. vetsuccess.gov/

Family Services

National Guard Family Program—Quickly find national, state, and local veteran and family-related resources such as: Family Assistance Centers, military, health, child and youth resources. www.guardfamily.org/

Soldier Family Assistance Handbook—sfac.wramc.amedd.army.mil/Support/Handbooks/A%20Guide%20for%20Families%20of%20Wounded%20Soldiers.pdf

Defense and Veterans Brain Injury Center—www.dvbic.org/

Military HOMEFRONT—www.militaryhomefront.dod.mil/portal/page/itc/MHF/MHF_HOMEPAGE

Army Long-Term Family Case Management—https://www.hrc.army.mil/site/active/tagd/cmaoc/altfcm/index.htm

Fisher House—www.fisherhouse.org/

Battle mind—A buddy support website to help military personnel and families adjust from deployment to home life. www.battlemind.army.mil/

Veteran Service Officers Organizations

www.vfw.org—Veterans of Foreign Wars
www.amvets.org—American Veterans
www.dav.org—Disabled American Veterans
www.pva.org—Paralyzed Veterans of America
www.purpleheart.org—Military Order of the Purple Heart
www.legion.org—American Legion

www.nasdva.net—National Association of State Directors of Veterans Affairs

www.themilitarycoalition.org/Members.htm—Military Coalition Members

Tricare

www.tricare.mil—Tricare

www.tricaredentalprogram.com—Tricare Dental

www.trdp.org—Tricare Retiree Dental

www.healthnetfederalservices.com—Tricare North Region

www.humana-military.com—Tricare South Region

www.triwest.com—Tricare West Region

www.dmdc.osd.mil/appj/esgr/privacyaAction.do—Guard and Reserve Web portal to access for signing up for Tricare Reserve Select

www.tricare.mil/tma/MMSO/index.aspx—Military Medical Support Office (MMSO)

www.addp-ucci.com—Active Duty Dental Program

www.express-scripts.com—Tricare Pharmacy

Wounded Warrior Service Programs

www.aw2.army.mil—Army Wounded Warrior Program

www.m4l.usmc.mil—Marine for Life

www.npc.navy.mil/CommandSupport/SafeHarbor—Navy Safe Harbor—for Severely Injured Support

www.woundedwarrior.af.mil—Air Force Wounded Warrior Program

Organizations Specific to Disability

www.bva.org—Blind Veterans Association

www.nationalamputation.org—National Amputation Foundation

www.dvbic.org—Defense and Veterans Brian Injury Center

www.monkeyhelpers.org—Helping Hands

www.cdhs.state.co.us/tbi/definition_of_tbi.htm—Colorado Traumatic Brain Injury Trust Fund Program

www.operationtbifreedom.org—Denver Options—Operation TBI Freedom

Vacations for Wounded Service Members

www.vacationsforveterans.org—Vacations for Veterans (is to enable veterans of the United States Armed Forces recently wounded in combat operations and who has received the Purple Heart Medal in the Afghanistan or Iraq Campaigns to receive free lodgings donated by vacation homeowners)

Counseling

www.onefreedom.org—One Freedom
www.sunriseseminars.com—Sunrise Seminars
www.peoplehouse.org—People House
www.veteransandfamilies.org—Veterans and Families Coming Home
www.lostandfoundinc.org—Lost and Found Inc.
www.vets4vets.us—Vets 4 Vets
www.vhvnow.org—Veterans Helping Veterans Now
www.ppbhg.org—Pikes Peak Behavioral Health Group
www.annewein.com—Sleep Recover and Reintegration
www.artofredirection.com—Art of Redirection Counseling
www.giveanhour.org—Give an Hour
www.thesoldiersproject.org—Soldiers Project

Special Programs for OEF/OIF Wounded

www.challengeaspen.com—Challenge Aspen
www.challengedathletes.org—Challenged Athlete Foundation
www.dsusa.org—Disabled Sports USA
www.svasp.org—Sun Valley Adaptive Sports
www.independencefund.org—Independence Fund
www.sentinelsoffreedom.org—Sentinels of Freedom—Scholarships
www.operationfirstresponse.org—Operation First Response
www.woundedmarinecareers.org—Wounded Marine Careers Foundation
www.supportourwounded.org—Angels of Mercy
www.sentinelsoffreedom.org—Sentinels of Freedom
www.semperfifund.org—Semper Fi Fund (must be a Marine or been attached to a Marine unit on deployment when injuries took place)
www.operationfamilyfund.org—Operation Family Fund
www.pentagonfoundation.org—Pentagon Foundation
www.saluteheroes.org—Coalition to Salute America's Heroes
www.injuredmarinesfund.org—Family and Friends for Freedom Fund, Inc.
www.rebuildhope.org—Rebuild Hope
www.heartsandhorses.org—Hearts and Horses
www.pptrc.org—Pikes Peak Therapeutic Riding Center

www.cadenceriding.org—Cadence Riding
www.trectrax.org—Therapeutic Riding and Education Center
www.outdoorbuddies.org—Outdoor Buddies
www.woundedwarriorproject.org—Wounded Warrior Project
www.woundedheroesfund.net—Wounded Heroes Fund
operationimpact.ms.northropgrumman.com—Northup Grumman—assisting with employment
www.operationfamilyfund.org—Operation Family Fund
www.operationfirstresponse.org—Operation First Response
www.lakeshore.org—Lakeshore Foundation
www.tirrfoundation.org—Project Victory
www.woundedwarriorresourcecenter.com—Military OneSource Wounded Warrior Resource Center
www.strikeoutsfortroops.org—Strikeouts for Troops
www.hopeforthewarriors.org—Hope for the Warriors
remind.org—Bob Woodruff Foundation
www.injuredmarinesfund.org—Family and Friends for Freedom Fund
www.fisherhouse.org—Fisher House
www.transitionassistanceprogram.com—Wounded, Ill, and Injured Compensation and Benefits Handbook

Family Assistance

www.snowballexpress.org—Snowball Express
www.militaryonesource.com—Military OneSource
www.military.com—Military news with benefit information
www.freedomcalls.org—Freedom Calls
www.ssa.gov—Social Security
www.herosalute.com—Hero Salute
www.hrc.army.mil/site/active/tagd/cmaoc/altfcm/index.htm—Army Long-Term Family Case
www.nmfa.org—National Military Family Association
www.operationhomefront.org—Specific to Illinois
www.ourmilitary.mil/index.aspx—Our Military
www.uso.org—United Services Organization
www.cellphonesforsoldiers.com—Cell phones/calling cards for soldiers
www.homesforourtroops.org—Homes for Our Troops
www.rebuildingtogether.org—Rebuilding Together
www.soldiersangels.com—Soldiers Angels
www.taps.org—Tragedy Assistance Program for Survivors
www.nationalresourcedirectory.org—National Resource Directory

www.armedforcesfoundation.org—Armed Forces Foundation

www.veteransholidays.com—Veterans Holidays (discounted rates)

www.swords-to-plowshares.org—Swords to Plowshares (Employment, Training, Health, and Legal)

www.grandcamps.org—Grand Camps for kids and grandparents

www.myarmyonesource.com—Army One Source

www.chooselifeinc.org—Assistance with resume, job readiness training, etc.

www.projectsanctuary.us—Project Sanctuary

www.freedomhunters.org—Freedom Hunters

www.redcross.org—American Red Cross

www.emilitary.org—The Military Family Network

www.focusproject.org—Project Focus

www.militaryhomefront.dod.mil—Military HOMEFRONT

www.militarystudent.org—Military Students on the Move

www.military.com/spouse—Military Spouse Career Center

www.naccrra.org—National Association of Child Care Resource and Referral Agencies

www.milspouse.org—Military Spouse Resource Center—assist with employment, education, scholarships

www.fns.usda.gov/wic—Women, Infants, and Children (WIC)

www.ourmilitarykids.org—Our Military Kids

Financial Assistance

www.reserveaid.org—Reserve Aid

www.unmetneeds.com—Unmet needs

www.impactahero.org/index.php—Impact a Hero

www.saluteheroes.org—Salute Heroes for Wounded Warriors

www.thehomefrontcares.org—Home Front Cares

www.usacares.org—USA Cares

www.operationhomefront.net—Operation Home Front

www.soldierfoundation.org—American Soldier Foundation

www.AMF100.org—American Military Family

www.legion.org/veterans/family/assistance—American Legion Temporary Financial Assistance (TFA)

www.naavets.org—National Association of American Veterans

www.nvf.org/contact/rfs/index.php—National Veterans Foundation

www.helpingheal.org/guidelines.html—Operation Helping Healing

www.elks.org—Elks Lodge—have financial assistance available

Veterans Affair Programs

www.va.gov—Veteran Affairs
www.vetbiz.gov—Veteran Business
www.taapmo.com—Transition Assistant Advisor
www.va.gov/hac/forbeneficiaries/champva/champva.asp—CHAMPVA
for dependents

Transportation

www.veteransairlift.org—Veterans Airlift Command
www.aircompassionamerica.org—Air Ambulance Service
www.aircharitynetwork.org—Air Charity Network
www.angelflightwest.org—Angel Flight West
www.heromiles.org—Operation Hero Miles
www.mercymedical.org/helpful-links/—Mercy Medical

Employment

www.return2work.org—Return 2 Work
www.militaryconnection.com—Military Connection
www.vetjobs.com—Vet Jobs
www.hireamericasheroes.org—Hire Americas Heroes
www.helmetstohardhats.org—Helmets to Hardhats
www.enableamerica.org—Enable America
www.veteransgreenjobs.org—Veterans Green Jobs
www.americasheroesatwork.gov—Americas Heroes at Work
www.VetsJobs.net—Veteran Job Fairs
www.usajobs.gov—USA Jobs
www.hireAhero.com—Hire a Hero
www.hirevetsfirst.gov—Hire Vets First
www.MOAA.org—Military Officers Association of America
www.RecruitArmy.com—Recruit Army
www.recruitnavy.com—Recruit Navy
www.recruitairforce.com—Recruit Airforce
www.recruitmarines.com—Recruit Marines
www.5starrecruitment.com—5 Star Recruitment Career
acp-usa.org—American Corporate Program—Veterans Mentoring
www.460fss.com/460_FSS/HTML/HRO.html—Buckley AFB NAF Human Resource Office
www.coloradoworkforce.com—Colorado Department of Labor and Employment

regionalhelpwanted.com/colorado-springs-jobs—Colorado Springs Help Wanted

www.jobsearch.org—Job Bank

www.gssa.state.co.us/announce/Job+Announcements.nsf/ $about?OpenAbout—Colorado State Government Job Announcements

Military

www.archives.gov—National Archives and Records Administration

www.dmdc.osd.mil/rsl/owa/home—DEERS/RAPIDS Locator

www.themilitarycoalition.org—Military Coalition

www.transitionassistanceprogram.com—Transition Assistance Program Turbo Tap

www.militaryaudiology.org—Military Audiology

www.OnetCenter.org—To transfer Military Occupation Specialty to Civilian

Education/Scholarships

www.fishhouse.org—Fish House Foundation

www.cfsrf.org—Children of Fallen Heroes

www.freedomalliance.org—Freedom Alliance

www.militaryscholar.org—Scholarships for military children

www.dantes.doded.mil—Troops to teachers

Service Specific

www.npc.navy.mil—Navy Personnel Command

www.afcrossroads.com—Air Force Cross Roads

www.hrc.army.mil/indexflash.asp—U.S. Army Human Resource Command

www.marines.mil/Pages/Default.aspx—Marines

www.uscg.mil—U.S. Coast Guard

Service Specific Financial Assistance

www.afas.org—Air Force Aid Society (AFAS), they also have a loan called the Falcon loan which is $500 or less for emergency needs.

www.aerhq.org—Army Emergency Relief

www.cgmahq.org—Coast Guard Mutual Assistance (Active, Reserve, and Retired)

www.nmcrs.org—Navy-Marine Corps Relief Society Financial Assistance

Housing

www.homesforourtroops.org—Home for Our Troops—(they will build you a house at no cost if accepted)

www.buildinghomesforheroes.com—Building Homes for Heroes

www.rebuildingtogether.org—Rebuilding Together believes we can preserve affordable homeownership and revitalize communities by providing free home modifications and repairs, making homes safer, more accessible, and more energy efficient.

www.operationforeverfree.org—Operation Forever Free

Legal

www.nvlsp.org—National Veterans Legal Services Program

www.abanet.org—American Bar Association, Pro Bono Programs (information on free legal services)

NATIONAL INFORMATION CENTER FOR CHILDREN AND YOUTH WITH DISABILITIES

PO Box 1492
Washington, DC 20013

NATIONAL TOLL-FREE NUMBERS

A

AIDS Factline	800-662-6080
Academy of Dentistry for Persons with Disabilities	800-621-8099
Alliance of Genetic Support Groups	800-342-2348
Alzheimer's Diseases & Related Disorders	800-621-0379
AMC Cancer Information & Counseling Line	800-525-3777
American Association on Mental Retardation	800-424-3688
American Cancer Society	800-227-2345
American Cleft Palate Educational Foundation	800-242-5338
American College of Allergy & Immunology	800-842-7777
American Council for the Blind	800-424-8666
American Diabetes Association National Service Center	800-232-3472
American Federation of Teachers	800-238-1133
American Foundation for the Blind	800-232-5463

American Kidney Foundation.. 800-638-8299
American Kidney Fund...800 638-8299
American Liver Foundation.. 800-223-0179
American Lupus Society... 800-331-1802
American Paralysis Association 800-225-0292
American Speech-Language-Hearing Association............... 800-638-8255
American Trauma Society 800-556-7890
American Tuberous Sclerosis Association........................... 800-446-1211
Apple Office of Special Education (Disability Solutions).... 800-732-3131
Association of Heart Patients Helpline.............................. 800-241-6993

B

Better Hearing Institute Helpline... 800-424-8576
Blind Children's Center... 800-222-3566

C

Cancer Information Service National Line........................... 800-422-6237
Captioned Films for the Deaf.. 800-237-6213
"Careline" Information & Referral....................................... 800-662-7030
Center for Special Education Technology............................ 800-345-8322
Children's Defense Fund 800-424-9602
Children's Hospice International... 800-242-4453
CLEFT Palate Foundation 800-242-5338
Close Look LD Teen Line... 800-522-3458
Cornelia de Lange Syndrome Foundation............................ 800-223-8355
Cystic Fibrosis Foundation.. 800-344-4823
Cystic Fibrosis Research Hotline 800-824-5064

D

D. T. Watson Rehabilitation Hospital 800-223-8806
Drug Abuse Hotline... 800-544-5437

E

Educators Publishing Service, Inc. for Specific
    Learning Disability 800-225-5750
Epilepsy Foundation of America.. 800-332-1000
Epilepsy Information Line.. 800-426-0660

ERIC Clearinghouse on Adult Career & Vocational ED...... 800-848-4815

F

Federation of Families for Children's Mental Health 800-969-6642
Federal Hill-Burton Free Care Program 800-492-0359
Financial Aid for Education Available from the
    Federal Government 800-638-6833

H

Handicapped Media, Inc. 800-321-8708
Hansen Disease (Leprosy) 800-543-3131
Health Care Financing Administration 800-492-6603
Hearing Aid Helpline 800-521-5247
Higher Education & the Handicapped (HEATH) 800-544-3284
Human Growth Foundation for Growth Disorders 800-451-6434

I

IBM National Support Center for Persons
    with Disabilities 800-426-2133
Information Center for Special Education
    Media & Materials 800-772-7372
International Craniofacial Foundation 800-535-3643
International Shriners Headquarters 800-237-5055

J

Job Accommodation Network (JAN) 800-526-7234
Job Opportunities for the Blind (JOB) 800-638-7518
John Tracey Clinic on Deafness 800-522-4582
Juvenile Diabetes Foundation International 800-223-1138

L

Let's Play to Grow 800-224-7529
Little People America 800-243-9273
Living Bank-Organ Donors 800-528-2971
Lung Line (Lung Disorders, Allergies) 800-222-5864
Lupus Foundation of America 800-558-0121

M

Mainstream Information Center 800-223-2711

N

National Adolescent Suicide Hotline 800-621-4000
National Adoption Center... 800-862-3678
National Association for Hearing & Speech Action 800-638-8255
National Association for Parents for the
    Visually Impaired 800-561-6265
National Association for Retarded Citizens
    of the U.S. 800-433-5255
National Association for Sickle Cell Diseases, Inc. 800-421-8453
National Cancer Institute Information Service...................... 800-422-6237
National Captioning Institute.. 800-321-8337
National Center for Missing & Exploited Children 800-843-5678
National Center for Stuttering 800-221-2483
National Center for the Prevention of Sudden
    Infant Death Syndrome... 800-638-7437
National Center for Youth with Disabilities......................... 800-333-6293
National Clearinghouse for Alcohol & Drug
    Information 800-662-4357
National Committee for Citizens in Education 800-638-9675
National Crisis Center for the Deaf...................................... 800-446-9876
National Cystic Fibrosis Foundation 800-344-4823
National Down Syndrome Congress 800-232-6372
National Down Syndrome Society 800-221-4602
National Easter Seals Society 800-221-6827
National Eye Care Project Hotline 800-222-3937
National Foundation of Dentistry for the
    Handicapped 800-873-3335
National Fragile X Foundation 800-688-8765
National Head Injury Foundation
    (Patients & Family only) 800-444-6443
National Health Information Center (NHIC) 800-336-4797
National Hearing Aid Society.. 800-521-5247
National Information Center for Children &
    Youth with Disabilities... 800-999-5599
National Information Center for Educational Media............. 800-421-8711
National Information Systems for Health Related Services 800-922-9234

National Information Center for Orphan Drugs &
  Rare Diseases 800-336-4797
National Information Center on Deaf/Blindness 800-672-6720
National Jewish Center for Immunology &
  Respiratory Medicine 800-222-5864
National Kidney Foundation, Inc. 800-622-9010
National Liberty Services for the Blind &
  Physically Handicapped 800-424-8567
National Multiple Sclerosis Society 800-822-3379
National Organization on Disability 800-248-2253
National Organization for Rare Disorders (NORD) 800-477-6673
National Parkinson Foundation 800-327-4545
National Rehabilitation Information Center 800-346-2742
National Retinitis Pigmentosa Foundation 800-638-2300
National Reye's Syndrome Foundation 800-233-7393
National Runaway Switchboard 800-621-4000
National Secondary Surgical Opinion Program 800-638-6833
National Spinal Cord Injury Association 800-962-9629
National Spinal Cord Injury Hotline 800-526-3456
National Society to Prevent Blindness 800-331-2020
National Sudden Infant Death Syndrome Foundation 800-221-7437
National Tuberous Sclerosis Association, Inc. 800-225-6872

O

Occupational Hearing Services (OHS) 800-222-3277
Office of Health Promotion & Disease Prevention
  Health Information Center 800-336-4797
Office of Minority Health Resource Center 800-444-6472
Orton Dyslexia Society 800-222-3123

P

Parents Anonymous Hotline 800-421-0353
Parents Resource Institute for Drug Education (PRIDE) 800-221-9746
Parkinson's Education Program 800-344-7877
Practitioner's Reporting System for Medical Services 800-638-6725

R

RP Foundation Fighting Blindness 800-638-2300

Runaway Hotline 800-231-6946

S

Simmon's Foundation for Continence................................. 800-237-4666
Social Security Administration 800-234-5772
Special Education Software Center 800-327-5892
Spina Bifida Hotline 800-621-3141
Sturge-Weber Foundation 800-627-5482
Stuttering Foundation of America 800-992-9392
Sudden Infant Death Syndrome Alliance 800-638-7437

T

Tele-Consumer Hotline.. 800-332-1124
Terri Gotthelf Lupus Research Institute 800-825-8787
Tourette Syndrome Association 800-237-0717
Tripod-Grapevine Service for Hearing Impaired 800-352-8888

U

United Cerebral Palsy Association, Inc. (UCPA) 800-872-1827
U.S. Government TDD Directory 800-877-8339

Index

About the Authors

Janelle Hill is presently the president and lead consultant of PBSM/Federal Concierge, LLC and director of the Federal Capital Planning & Investment Control Forum. Janelle serves as an advisor and consultant in the arenas of marketing, business development, and sales in the government. Janelle works directly for Chief Information Officer Program Management Offices, directing and supporting senior management with their portfolio management, information technology (security), and capital planning investment initiatives.

Janelle has written extensively; producing white papers, all facets of proposal support, technical requirements, Capital Asset business case justifications, Capital Portfolio Investment Control documents, and a variety of governance documentation products for congressional reviews. Through her love of writing, a contractor assignment at the Department of Veterans Affairs and several years experience of being a former military wife, Janelle identified a number of challenges unique to military and Veterans' transitional and family issues. Through this inspiration, Janelle teamed up with Don Philpott to coauthor the *Capital Planning & Investment Control Guidebook* and the *Wounded Warriors Handbook* ("The Red Book"). Now Janelle, Don, and Cheryl Lawhorne have teamed up for the *Military Marriage Manual* and are continuing to grow the Rowan & Littlefield Military Life Series of publications.

Don Philpott is the editor-in-chief of *International Homeland Security: The Quarterly Journal for Homeland Security Professionals* and the author of more than 5,000 articles in various publications and over 100 books, including *The Wounded Warrior Handbook* (2008), *Is America Safe?* (2009), *The Military Marriage Manual* (2010), *Combat-Related Traumatic Brain Injury* *and PTSD* (2010), and *A Guide to Federal Terms and Acronyms* (2010). He lectures on security and communications and is a regular contributor to radio and television programs on security and other issues.